BECOMING A

Bedside Advocate

Insight & Information
to help your loved one through the
Modern Healthcare Experience

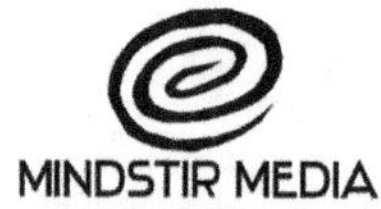

BECOMING A

Bedside Advocate

Insight & Information
to help your loved one through the
Modern Healthcare Experience

Kimberley Norris

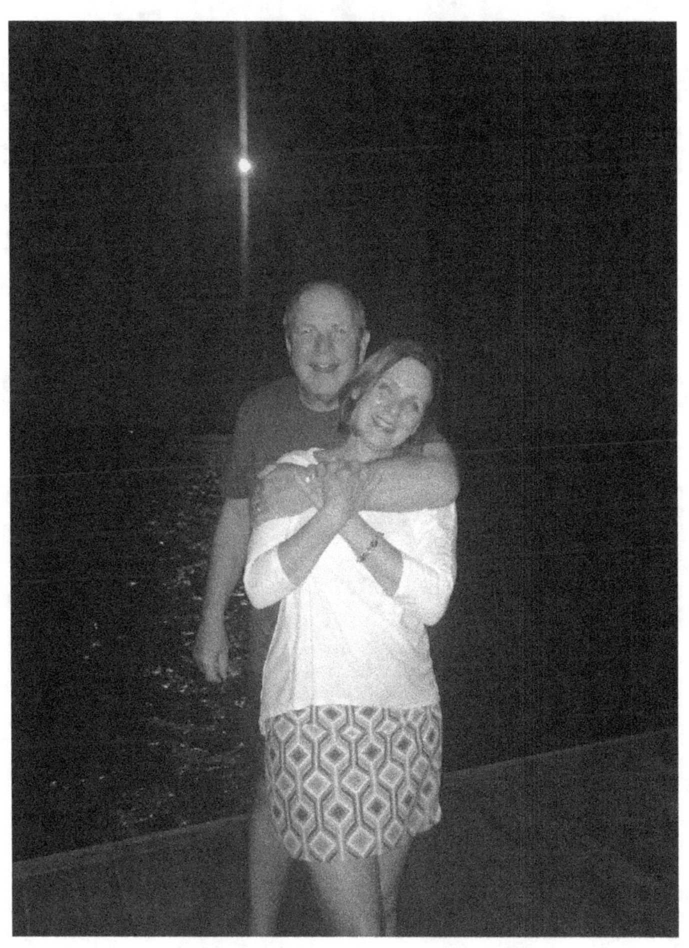

For Rick, our knight in shining armor.

Advocate:

One who pleads another's cause,
who helps another, by defending or comforting him.

Contents

CHAPTER ONE

Why I Wrote This Book

My husband of 32 years, Rick Norris, died of acute respiratory failure in December of 2018 as a result of Stage III esophageal cancer. His health ordeal lasted one year from diagnosis to death. I began writing this book in March 2019 to share my journey as his bedside advocate, with the aim of helping others who may one day find themselves in a similar position—a statistical probability as our loved ones age.

For us, Rick's health crisis came out of the blue. Though he initially showed no symptoms at all, he became one of over eight million seniors hospitalized in 2018. As anyone would be, our family was caught off guard—shocked. Our adult children and I were unequipped for the experiences to come—for the nature of the work ahead. There was no support system or guide book available to prepare us for our role as bedside advocates.

Over the eight weeks Rick spent in Duke University Hospital's cardiothoracic intensive care unit, I'd glimpse inside other rooms as I made my way down the corridors. They were filled with critically ill patients. Whether there for a heart transplant, a double lung transplant, or an esophagectomy, the patients were often accompanied by their spouses, sons, daughters, and lifelong family friends—enduring suffering alongside their loved ones.

I suspect these family members felt much like me, blindsided and overwhelmed, trying to make sense of the chaos and not sure how to comfort the people they hold so dear.

The medical professionals orbiting my husband's care were unbelievably dedicated, hardworking and brilliant. They were laser-focused on healing and saving my husband's life to the best of their ability, delivering sound medical care.

Medical caregiver-patient relationships are of primary importance, including during hospitalization. But the bedside advocate is also an integral part of patient care and recovery. There is no substitute—not even a trained professional—for the bond that families and lifelong friends have with one another. The connection arises from *love*, and that means years of intimate knowledge about the patient that cannot be gained in brief encounters with medical professionals in a hospital setting. This bond brings a level of awareness that can be valuable to the medical team and become an integral part of the care plan. For example, this profound insight may allow an engaged bedside advocate to be first to observe meaningful changes in the patient. A communicative advocate might offer information about the patient's baseline behavior that the physician can use to tailor treatment.

DEFINING THE "ADVOCATE"

> Advocatus (Latin): one called to aid another, a witness, supporter, mediator.

The bedside advocate role can be a life-changing, rewarding experience for you. To serve another—give protection and comfort, and to stand alongside another in need—is deeply within us all. The work can create deep fulfillment and growth. In many cases it can be a powerful gift: the last, precious opportunity to demonstrate devotion and to comfort your loved ones, bringing a sense of peace should they pass on. Because of the chaos that too often comes with critical illness, hospitalization, and the recovery process, being a proactive, compassionate advocate can help ground you and those around you during the disarray.

The better prepared we are, the more we harmoniously collaborate with caregivers, the wider the ripple effect that benefits everyone involved.

Perhaps surprisingly, however, bedside advocates are not always seen as helpful by hospitalists, attending physicians, surgeons and nurses. I interviewed several such professionals for this book, and while all are dedicated to doing their very best, there was at times an unfortunate undercurrent of "us vs. them" or even a hint of disdain in conversations about advocates —sometimes seemingly as a matter of fact and sometimes inadvertently. For some clinicians, there may even be an unspoken sense of dread when a family member is described as "advocate." Are they going to be a time and energy drain on the medical care team?

I want to help others understand that the relationship can be harmonious and beneficial to all—patients and families, and caregivers alike.

The goals of this book are simple: to establish that the bedside advocate is an important part of health care, and, to support and humanize that role by sharing my lessons learned through information, insight and perspective from the medical care team on the ground.

In this book, physicians and nurses tell us how they define a helpful bedside advocate. I came to understand this as good coaching, and I hope that my readers will benefit from their advice.

Without a doubt, the hospitalized patient will be better served when the medical care team—physicians, nurses, physical therapists, hospice care givers, discharge case managers—welcomes the advocate into patient-care relationship. The reality is that this invitation must be earned by the advocate, sometimes referred to as the "civilian." In a nutshell, that's why I wrote this book: so that you, and that all of us collectively, can become well-informed assets working in partnership with medical teams for the sake of the people we love.

WHAT ARE THE CHANCES THAT YOU'LL FIND YOURSELF IN THIS ROLE?

The most likely bedside advocates will come from America's largest adult population segments, which are 72.1 million Millennials (born 1981-1996) and their elders, 71.6 million Baby Boomers (born 1946-1964). That's 143.7 million of us. (Source: Pew Research Center, *Millennials over take Baby Boomers as America's largest generation,* reported April 28, 2020.)

In 2018 there were 52 million people aged 65 and older in the United States. Health care studies show in that same year nearly 17% of the 52 million elders were hospitalized. Predictably, the elderly account for the largest share of admissions in the U.S. Keep in mind that the number of hospitals has decreased in recent years although the country faces an increasing elder population.

In other words, in 2018 about 8 million elders were hospitalized within a landscape of perhaps overcrowded hospitals. I'm sure that in many cases, their spouses and adult children were called in to duty as advocates without any preparation. That is exactly what happened to our family, and the high likelihood that so many others in our society will one day face such a situation is increasingly clear.

THREE REASONS A BEDSIDE ADVOCATE IS CRITICAL FOR THE HOSPITALIZED PATIENT

Varun Verma, M.D., former CEO of Medofi, published in 9/14/2018, *Patients need an advocate at the bedside* on KevinMD.com:

"The simple truth is that there is a pervasive "profits over patients" ethos in modern medicine that contributes to suboptimal patient care regardless of institution. Health care professionals constantly find themselves overworked and understaffed, and their employers seem to get away with this *because despite health care being a heavily regulated industry, there is no oversight of the moment-to-moment management of patients.*"

Dr. Verma clarifies that bedside patient advocates are critical because they will:

1. help the patient remember to address their concerns

2. provide valuable information to the medical team

3. foster more engagement from the medical team by knowing that the patient and caregivers have a valuable trusted ally at the bedside.

The better informed they are, the better bedside advocates can cope and serve their loved ones. For civilians like myself, it often starts with having the big picture in mind—knowing *how* and *when* to ask the right questions and share information; digesting the information we receive within our own limitations; and figuring out how best to partner with care teams.

CHAPTER TWO

What Happened to Rick

Each of us will have our own unique experience when coping with a health crisis. Your journey will be different from mine. But there are some things, certain lessons learned, that when shared by one another can benefit everyone. That is what I hope to accomplish with this book: to share the lessons I wish I'd known before it all started.

We were living in New Jersey… a happy, fortunate life, but not without our share of challenges and hard work. In May of 2016, following our daughter's wedding in North Carolina, we set out for a weekend retreat in Palmetto Bluff, located in Bluffton, South Carolina. Palmetto Bluff is a destination and conservancy in South Carolina's exquisite low country by the May River—home to water fowl and alligators… abundant wild game… bald eagles and bluebirds… graceful live oaks hundreds of years old… the May River and its magical dolphins… and laid-back, comforting, Southern charm. Quite a change from our 30-year work life in the New York metropolitan area!

On one glorious, cloudless low-country day, we leisurely drove through the town, and it took just a few minutes for the spell to be cast: We fell in love with South Carolina.

By Labor Day weekend, we'd signed a two-year lease on a house in a neighborhood within walking distance of the river and moved away from our New Jersey life with a sense of adventure.

Suddenly, our world was completely different. We thought perhaps we might retire in this magical place. The stay in the rental house on Myrtle View Street felt like a vacation. Our second-floor bedroom had French doors that opened onto a porch that was canopied by trees. We threw open the doors at night to enjoy the fresh air and awoke each day wonderfully rested. It was like "sleeping in a huge treehouse," we whispered to one another in the night.

The house was an easy walk to the community dock on the May River, considered to be a treasure of coastal South Carolina. It was a treat to be able to walk down to the serene, graceful river, especially at dusk with a cocktail in hand, sometimes with a few lovely neighbors, to watch the dolphins and waterfowl.

Both of us enjoyed the river, but Rick in particular. He started fishing a little off the dock and casting the net for shrimp with encouragement from our neighbor Stan. He delighted in riding bikes, swimming, kayaking and oyster roasts. There were lovely establishments within walking distance for cocktails, a bite to eat and conversation with interesting patrons. We started to make friends who would join us on short notice for neighborhood dinners and conversation, making us feel at home.

We loved the Bluffton area, with Savannah's charm just a short drive away. We agreed it was time to begin looking for a small retirement home to buy ... blissfully ignorant of what was to come.

It was a year later, November of 2017. I was having my annual physical, and Rick sat in the waiting room, bored. He happened to pick up a pamphlet that said if you're of a certain age, were ever a smoker and have a history of melanoma, you should have a CT scan. So, pamphlet in hand, Rick walked into our doctor's office and set it up.

The CT scan came back showing a mass in his upper right lung. Our physician ordered a PET scan. The mass in the right lung turned out to be benign, but there was something showing in the esophagus. His gastroenterologist scheduled an endoscopy to look at and biopsy the esophagus. Rick had had decades of indigestion, but nothing bad enough for any of his doctors to make a big deal about other than to prescribe a medication.

His diagnosis was stage IIIA distal esophageal adenocarcinoma. No symptoms. No warning. This was just before Christmas of 2017.

According to the oncologist, we "lucked out." Another six months and Rick probably would have been Stage IV and would have been "kept comfortable." But now he was a candidate for treatment.

The gastroenterologist and oncologist recommended radiation and chemotherapy for six weeks, then surgery. An esophagectomy is complex major surgery to remove the esophagus and part of the stomach and requires an experienced specialist. Esophagus cancer, treatment and surgery are brutal, we were told.

We were slightly paralyzed. But, with the help of physicians and friends we were fortunate enough to find a good hospital for Rick's surgery.

Dr. D'Amico, chief of thoracic surgery at Duke University Hospital, came highly recommended as both a surgeon and "a gentleman." Exactly what we needed.

Again, we were fortunate that Duke Medical Center in Durham, North Carolina, is only a thirty-minute drive from the Raleigh home of our daughter Kelly and her husband, Stephen. It was important to have local family support, we were counseled.

On March 20, 2018, we drove the five hours from South Carolina to Durham and met Dr. D'Amico and his physician assistant, Scott Balderson. Dr. D'Amico was a slim, soft-spoken, self-assured man. Scott, warm and talkative. They seemed confident, and we felt confident enough in them. We asked a few questions, but we really did not know what to ask.

"How is pain managed?" Rick asked.

"No problem," we were assured. "There is a pain management team. We know how to handle it. Expect discomfort, yes, but pain we can handle."

We braced ourselves for what we expected to be a difficult surgery and a three-week hospital stay.

Rick had his esophagectomy at Duke University Hospital on April 16, 2018. He was critically ill and ended up staying in the ICU for eight weeks. After eleven weeks, on July 3, 2018, he was discharged to Encompass Health Rehabilitation Hospital of Bluffton, South Carolina, for another three weeks. There, he received excellent rehabilitative care to restore his body, frail from being bedridden and critically ill for so long. Finally, on July 20, he returned home to further recover, following what was nearly a fourteen-week hospitalization in all. And once home, he received continuous home care by an array of nurses, physical therapists, occupational therapists, speech therapists and custodial professionals.

He did recover enough to have almost three months at home to enjoy our neighborhood again. On September 26, 2018, Rick victoriously made the short walk to the neighborhood dock and at last enjoyed the beautiful May River he loved so much. He'd spoken of his return during the worst of times, half delirious in the hospital. "I want to go home ... I want to walk down to the dock ... When I get home, we're going to stop working and enjoy life more."

Then, in early October 2018, he began to have continuous episodes of pneumonia with constant ER visits and local hospitalizations. He lost a total of about 50 pounds by this time and couldn't keep foods or liquids down. He was starting to look emaciated, constantly suffering with respiratory failure, with bed sore wounds and weakness. We were blessed to have good medical care, home nursing, physical therapy and loving support from our neighbors and friends, but he was getting worse.

I reached out to the Duke surgeons in desperation, and my email was answered immediately. Scott Balderson, Dr. D'Amico's physician assistant, spoke with me by phone. They recommended Rick return to Duke to find the reasons for his complications.

In the midst of all this, our lease was due to run out on November 1, and the homeowners declined our request to extend the lease. Saying it was "now or never", Rick insisted that we try to buy a small home in the community we loved. It gave him a sense of well-being to accomplish our wish to retire there.

Within a week or so, we closed on a small house, trusted a local company to move our belongings, left with boxes stacked all over the new house, and drove the five hours to Duke to get Rick into the hospital again.

He was admitted on November 9 and sent home a week later. His surgery had healed nicely: The constant aspiration of digestive fluids into the lungs caused the pneumonia. We were on our own.

Rick's final hospitalization was from December 6 through 13, 2018, in nearby Savannah Memorial Hospital, where after spending three days in the ER, an ICU room opened. Then Rick went from the ICU to a step-down unit, where his respiratory failure could not be controlled. (A step-down unit is a hospital nursing unit providing care intermediately between that of an ICU and a normally staffed inpatient division.)

He was even more emaciated, calling out my name, occasionally reaching up with trembling arms extended to someone we couldn't see, like a child reaching up to a parent to be held. He suffered and fought to live. The doctors and nurses were compassionate but couldn't help him. He was dying, and aggressive measures to keep him alive were not only contrary to his end-of-life wishes, it would have been inhumane to push further. Then to hospice.

He mercifully passed on December 13, 2018, at 12:26 p.m. on Savannah Memorial Hospital's hospice floor.

He was in hospice less than twenty-four hours. Like many others, my husband used every ounce of his will and strength to try to stay with us. It was heart-wrenching—humbling—to witness. It brought our family and friends closer together.

When the ordeal of Rick's critical illness burst into our life, I knew zero about what to expect or how to protect and advocate for my husband. We had no idea how to navigate a hospital ICU or step-down units, rehabilitation, home care, critical ER visits or hospice. No notion of how important nurses were and how to work with the swirl of hospital caregivers. No true understanding of what ICU delirium was and how troubling it could be to witness.

Throughout this yearlong experience, I stumbled around and learned a great deal I'm eager to share. My hope is that you'll find the lessons I learned, and the insights offered by medical professionals, to be helpful should you face similar struggles one day. This book is for you.

CHAPTER THREE

Prepare for Battle

Once the reality of my husband's illness was revealed, what happened after wasn't a gradual thing. Critical events can happen quickly, as they did for us, or they may unfold over a longer period of time. Either way, having your affairs in order is a great advantage … though too many of us put it off.

I'm no legal or financial expert, but if it is within your ability to do so, being prepared with updated documents is the responsible thing to do.

THE IMPORTANCE OF HEALTH CARE DIRECTIVES

Rick and I forced ourselves to revisit the conversation about his end-of-life wishes. It was difficult, but doing so helped me advocate for Rick when the time came—in the emergency rooms and hospital units, and while in hospice service.

Along the way, an ER nurse coached me to carry a hard copy of the documents at all times. "You may never need them," she said, "but if you do, having the legal documents in hand will be very important."

She was right.

Just ten days before Rick died, we went from a small-town ER in the middle of the night to the chaos of a large, overcrowded

Savannah ER in one 15-hour period. But I had his medical records and documents in hand wherever we went, and it proved helpful.

Remember that each state may have different requirements, so it's important to seek legal advice where you are located. Here's a checklist of the basic legal documents to discuss with a lawyer. Even counsel through a service such as Legal Zoom can help:

- ✓ health care directives
- ✓ last will and testament
- ✓ health care power of attorney
- ✓ do-not-resuscitate directive

MEDICAL INSURANCE

First let me say this: Insurance can be an enormous issue for the advocate, as navigating the nuances of health care coverage in the U.S. is an intricate endeavor. Whether privately insured, uninsured, underinsured, Medicaid or Medicare coverage, you may face any number of complexities, such that I am not qualified to competently address.

This I do know for certain: Whatever your health care insurance circumstances, it's best to take time to understand your coverage or lack thereof.

If you have health care insurance, there is no time like the present to review your policy with your agent or carrier so that you'll be clear about your coverage. Even if you *think* you know what is covered, do an in-depth review anyway.

If you are uninsured or underinsured, find out as much as you can and discuss it with the hospital. The more you know, the better you can navigate the billing.

Because the minutiae of insurance coverage can be difficult to remember in the moment, it may be helpful to record your conversations when speaking by phone with a carrier or agent—with their permission, of course. I have yet to have a medical professional or agent decline to be recorded when I explained it was for my notes only. Once it's recorded, you can transcribe the important parts of the conversation in hard-copy notes to use as reference or to file away. I used a Sony digital voice recorder and a Sony compact-style earphone microphone to easily record phone conversations on my iPhone—again, only with the explicit permission from the people on the calls.

Predicting hospitalization costs is very difficult because, obviously, charges are not really known until the billing is done. But if you're aware of your coverage, charges can be effectively questioned, perhaps even negotiated, and you'll reduce the pressure of paying bills that may be incorrectly coded. Here are some other things to consider, based on my experience:

MEDICARE INSURANCE

Like most Boomers 65 and over, Rick was prepared with Medicare and Medicare Supplemental Insurance. This combined coverage saved us from having to pay deductibles and the 20% of cost not covered by Medicare. Without Medicare Supplemental insurance, we would have been left to struggle with a significant debt. The monthly premium for Medicare Supplemental coverage was minimal, and well worth the value to offset the potential additional costs. Medicare coverage and premiums can change each year, so please be sure to consult an insurance agent to understand your options.

INSURANCE COVERAGE FOR INPATIENT VS OUTPATIENT REHABILITATION

This can be important, because it is common to need either outpatient, nursing home or inpatient rehabilitation after a long hospitalization.

Inpatient rehabilitation coverage felt a little complicated, because we found it was based on how well Rick progressed over 21 days. Be sure to question and understand your insurance carrier's policies, Medicaid, Medicare or private insurance, specifically regarding inpatient rehabilitation. For me, speaking directly to an inpatient rehabilitation hospital administrator clarified exactly how the billing would work for Rick. If rehab is outpatient, coverage could be different, so it's important to ask questions about and understand outpatient vs. inpatient rehabilitation.

FINDING THE MEDICAL EXPERTS— JUST DO YOUR VERY BEST

Who really knows the best treatment or physician for your situation? One can conduct online research, and opinions are easy to find. In reality, the future can't be perfectly predicted. We can only do our best with the information available and take guidance from those who are knowledgeable.

In our case, hospitalization and major surgery were our path. Others will face different situations, but the sentiment above remains the same for everyone.

I learned this lesson: You've got to believe in your medical team. Once we made our decision and placed our trust in Dr. D'Amico of Duke Medical Center and his brilliant team, there could be no second guessing when times were brutal. Truthfully, I did have a lapse of faith in the decision for Rick's esophagectomy at one point during his recovery in Duke's ICU and got lost in desperation. It's a good teaching moment we'll talk about in another chapter.

To paraphrase Dr. Paul Speicher, many times with critical illness, there is no right answer, no supporting study, only the judgment and experience of the attending physician to trust. As, Dr. Danielle Ofri put it: "This is not an airplane repair."

Several times I reassured my fearful husband by saying things such as: "You're fortunate to be here at Duke Medical Center. The doctors and nurses are brilliant, and they're working hard to bring you home. We've got the best medical team in America. You're going to get better. Dr. D'Amico has seen it all. You're going to get better."

I was overwhelmed by Rick's suffering, but we had to believe that we'd done our very best to put his life in talented, dedicated hands. Of course, trust is to be earned and verified by actions, as observed by the bedside advocate. But once it's been attained, try to maintain that trust and faith. Otherwise there can be no peace.

Your medical team will do their very best to look after your loved one and engage with you as a responsible advocate. The reality is, medical professionals are human beings and are therefore imperfect, as we all are, but they're doing their very best.

Choosing Rick's Surgical Team

We started with seeking guidance from Rick's radiologist, oncologists and gastroenterologist. We listened and asked questions.

You'll never know who is in your extended social, community and professional network unless you reach out in all directions. Sometimes simple proximity, perhaps your immediate neighborhood, is everything. Sometimes your research will bring you to a particular physician you don't even know. Reach out … make the call … ask for help…be persistent.

Based on my experience, I wouldn't hesitate to travel to another city for the best care, as long as there is a friend or family support network with restful, temporary living space close by. In the likelihood that the next stage of treatment or surgery turns into a long, difficult ordeal as ours did, having the uplifting energy of true friends and loving family around will help both the patient and the advocate.

Questions in Preparation for Surgery or Hospitalization

The better the questions asked before surgery or treatment by the patient and advocate, the more your medical team will tell you. Many patients simply do not want to know much, and that is certainly understandable. But in the long run, I experienced that it was to the benefit of everyone involved to be on the same page with regard to recovery and expectations for quality of life.

When I interviewed Dr. D'Amico for this book, he noted that different surgeons will approach educating patients prior to surgery differently. They will abide by the ethics of surgery, discuss the nature, purpose, risks and benefits, pros and cons of the surgery, and answer your questions.

But where does the surgeon draw the line in sharing the possible risks? If a surgeon were to go through every risk and misery that can possibly happen, it would surely be too disturbing for many patients and, in some cases, may even become a self-fulfilling prophecy. This is sometimes referred to as the "nocebo effect," when negative symptoms occur in people because they expect them.

So, it's to the patient's and family advocate's benefit to bring up their deep concerns. How will pain-management work? What can we expect for quality of life? Is there risk of death from the procedure? There are plenty of people who simply do not want to know the details, and that's fine too.

Do your best to research the disease and treatment options. Every surgeon and ICU nurse I've interviewed recommended that the patient and family advocate research and learn as much as possible, as soon as possible, about the patient's disease, the surgery and recovery.

It's going to help immensely to gather information about the surgery and disease on your own. Try to digest why your loved one is in the hospital or having surgery to begin with. Start with a quick internet search for example. Then form your specific questions to ask your surgeon prior to surgery or hospitalization. The doctor and medical team will answer your concerns, but you must ask. It may feel surreal and painful to face but try your best to do it anyway.

In my case, I didn't ask enough questions up front about the complexity of the surgery and didn't have a realistic expectation of how brutal Rick's recovery could be, and that didn't help.

Answers to the few questions we did manage to ask up front strengthened my resolve when the worst did happen. I was able to say to myself, "Okay, we were told this might happen. This is to be expected."

QUESTIONS YOU MAY WANT TO ASK YOUR DOCTOR

- What are the best surgery or treatment options at this point?

- What is the risk/benefit to each option?

- What is the likelihood of survival from the disease if we do the less invasive vs. aggressive treatment or major surgery? What is the quality of life likely to be?

- What are the two or three most worrisome things that we should be prepared for during recovery from surgery?

CHAPTER FOUR

What the 'White Coats' Want You to Know

The "white coats"—the doctors and nurses who care for us—are the good guys entrusted with our lives and the lives of our loved ones. What's their perspective? How do they see the advocate?

I interviewed surgeons and hospitalists who were part of my husband's care, and one who was outside of our care experience. Each were asked, "What do you want patient advocates to know?" They all had a lot to say.

Physicians I happened to meet socially while writing this chapter, with little to no prompting, could not help themselves from sharing anecdotes of their frustration with the practice of medicine today. (Their stories supported the comments of the white coats I interviewed, but because my conversations with them were casual and "off the record," I didn't include them in this book.)

Off the record and on, the demands of electronic medical records (EMR) documentation were a recurring topic of conversation. It's not something civilians like myself would ordinarily be aware of, but it impacts hospital patient care a great deal, and it is causing burnout among medical professionals.

A December 31, 2019, *New York Times* article by Theresa Brown and Stephen Bergman titled "Doctors, Nurses and the Paperwork Crisis That Could Unite Them" made points that were repeatedly brought up by the physicians I interviewed. To quote the article:

> "Workloads have become heavier the last several years thanks almost entirely to the arrival of electronic health records—detailed reports about a patient's medical history and care. On average, nurses and doctors spend 50% of their work day treating the screen, not the patient, and that 'increased documentation time' associated with electronic health records can lead to burnout … The current system is pushing both doctors and nurses to the breaking point … [with] 44% of physicians feeling 'burned out.'"

Even more troubling are studies showing high suicide rates among doctors and nurses. Physicians have the highest suicide rate among all professions, according to the Medscape National Physician Burnout, Depression & Suicide Report 2019.

Similarly, nurses are seeing an increase in suicides, as shown in a study led by Judy Davidson, RN, DNP, of the University of California San Diego School of Medicine, and colleagues. The results of this research are published in the October 2019 *Archives of Psychiatric Nursing*.

In interviewing these caregivers, shifting my perspective from advocate to the physicians and nurses was very enlightening, and it seemed that it was almost cathartic for them. I came away with surprising insight and a couple of overarching points:

1. The advocate has to be responsible and ask the right questions if we want good information. That is difficult for civilians because so many things sabotage our ability to communicate and offer meaningful observation— lack of self-control, exhaustion, despair, ignorance, and grief among them.

2. The white coats, in general, think advocates can and should do a lot better and think we should be more aware and better informed than we are. They note that unprepared advocates can be so disruptive as to make physicians spend valuable time trying to communicate with those of us who aren't equipped. Few doctors or nurses want to waste time on confrontational, accusatory complainers. There is more information available to us now than ever before, and as advocates, we can always become better informed.

3. Many family advocates have unrealistic expectations of medicine, seeing it as an exact science, expecting perfection. The reality is that there is more gray area and we've got to be more comfortable with that.

As you read the comments from both physicians and nurses, try not to be overwhelmed. Responsibility can be shared with friends and family who are willing to help by advocating as a team. I would venture to say, in most hospitals, bedside advocates are in a tough position and need backup.

What follows are words of advice and perspective, some in direct quotes, others paraphrased and summarized, from several hours of face-to-face interviews regarding hospitalization. (Where paraphrased and summarized, I've done my best to neither water down nor inject my own point of view into their comments.) Not all hospitals are exactly alike, but they're close enough that I believe you'll find the white coats' information helpful.

These are the physicians and the nurse I interviewed and whose insight is shared:

THOMAS A. D'AMICO, MD
Gary Hock Endowed Professor of Surgery
Chief, Section of General Thoracic Surgery
Duke University Medical Center
Durham, North Carolina

PAUL J. SPEICHER, MD, MHS
Huntsville Cardiothoracic Surgeons
Huntsville, Alabama

DANIELLE OFRI, MD, PhD, D LITT (HON), FACP
Bellevue Hospital
NYU School of Medicine
Editor-in-Chief, Bellevue Literary Review
New York, New York

DWAYNE GARD, MD, CHIEF HOSPITALIST
Memorial University Medical Center
Savannah, Georgia

BETHLEHEM PETERS, RN, BSN
Cardiothoracic Intensive Care Unit
Duke University Medical Center
Durham, North Carolina

WHAT THE PHYSICIANS HAD TO SAY

The Big Picture of Hospitals:

Listening to physicians, both surgeons and hospitalists, I could not help but feel their frustration. It was a bit stunning at times because, like most people, I just couldn't see the bigger picture.

Comments from Dr. Danielle Ofri, whose sentiments were echoed in one way or another by the other physicians, set a backdrop for me:

"We often have expectations of medicine as an absolute science. You put in a value, make a calculation, and an outcome comes out the other end. But, it's not like that. There's a mix of judgment calls, prognosis and art on top of the science. There's much we don't know, and plenty of gray area. Patients can be upset and angry when they get an ambiguous response. But that is the reality. Every patient is different, and they don't fit into boxes the way textbooks say. Studies are done on populations and yield results that are an average. We don't know where you fit into that average so we can't give you an exact prognosis or treatment. Patients don't expect this, so some feel they have a terrible doctor. Trying to get comfortable with ambiguity is difficult. That's the way medicine is—ambiguous."

When I asked if this frustrated her, she told me, "It's just that I have to explain this over and over. Ambiguity is complicated to explain and it's very unsatisfying for the patient. It's very hard to explain why a test doesn't give a perfect answer and it takes a long time. It ends up taking away from all the other things I need to do for my patients."

Dr. Dwayne Gard, our hospitalist and hospice lead during my husband's final week of life in Savannah Memorial Health University Medical Center, made the observation that over the past ten years, aggressive behavior toward doctors and nurses has become more pronounced. And the hospital culture of downplaying employee abuse is pervasive.

He sees the aggression as a breakdown in communication that isn't necessarily the fault of patients and their families. Rather, it is a sign of a health care system that is already complex and becoming moreso, making it increasingly difficult for patients and their families to navigate the hospital system. And, Dr. Gard noted, hospital employees never know the kind of outside pressures the families are under, which might include drug addiction, insurance concerns, financial uncertainty or unemployment, to name just a few.

Then there is the daily, unattainable expectation that physicians should be perfect. Many doctors feel they are being asked to do the impossible in terms of patient care. There aren't enough minutes in an hour to effectively see all the patients and tackle all the electronic medical records.

Dr. Ofri pointed out, in no uncertain terms, that we ask of physicians a perfection that can't be humanly achieved. In fact, according to a Medscape.com article titled "Physicians Experience Highest Suicide Rate of Any Profession," there are many reasons for the numbers shown in the alarming research in which the piece is rooted.

In light of all of this, I asked Dr. Ofri if she was concerned that today's expectations of perfection will make medicine an unattractive profession. Her reply was encouraging:

"No. We still have 50,000 to 60,000 students applying to 18,000 spots in medical school. The people who went into medicine for money and prestige have long since decamped for Wall Street. It's a lot easier to make money there, and you don't have to do ten years of training or have people vomit on your shoes."

"The people who go into medicine now do it for the right reasons. They are compassionate, committed and dedicated to helping others. I worry, though, that the system wears them down. They get overwhelmed with electronic busy work and have more work than they can possibly do. For example, the physician has to check off that they've screened for domestic violence, depression, HIV, and they're all important, but there is not enough time for it. The system forces them to cut corners and, even lie. Making an ethical person do that is corrosive to the spirit."

Among Dr. Ofri's published works is a June 8, 2019, *New York Times* article that's an interesting read: "The Business of Health Care Depends on Exploiting Doctors and Nurses."

The impossible expectations and financial stressors of health care economics trickle down to the "boots on the ground," and those boots are filled by human beings in white coats.

I'm far from an expert on the topic of doctor and nurse burnout, and I certainly don't have the solution. But listening to the white coats and *how* they spoke was so valuable to me that I have to share their perspectives with you.

It's a part of the bigger health care picture I personally didn't know going into our experience. Certainly, during the stress of advocating for my critically ill husband, the very last thing on my mind was the burdens of the doctors and nurses, and they certainly didn't make it an issue or an excuse. But now I know that the pervasive expectation of unattainable perfection is part of their everyday reality.

We'd all agree, I'm sure, that we need brilliant, compassionate, dedicated doctors and nurses. Thank God that's exactly what my husband had at Duke Medical Center during his surgery and brutal recovery. I just wish I'd known their perspective before it all started, because it would have made me a better advocate.

How a Hospital Works:

Dr. Ofri's description of a hospital was easiest for me to digest:

"People have the impression that hospitals are straightforward, orderly places, but it's not like that at all. There are a million moving parts and people, and it can't be any other way. Every patient requires an enormous medical team because health care is so complex today. Every position has to be covered 24/7, and there will always be turnovers and changes. By definition, it's a complicated beehive."

Every single one of the doctors and nurses I interviewed completely understood that hospitalization is rough on us civilians. "Like you've parachuted onto Mars," as Dr. Ofri puts it. We civilians are disoriented and overwhelmed, don't know the language or the rules, and don't expect the inevitable chaos. We often go into survival mode, stunned by witnessing our loved ones' suffering and feeling the need to defend them.

We need coaching from the white coats on the inside.

From the Physicians

Tips for Advocates During Hospitalization

- Get a list identifying who is on your hospital team, such as your attending physician, hospitalist or fellow. Use an organizational chart. Go over it with someone on that team, and don't be afraid to say, "I just want to understand who's responsible for my loved one's care. Can you spend a minute or two with me on this org chart?" Refer to the chart when you need to communicate with a member of the medical team, and remember, there will be turnovers for night and weekend coverage. (See Figure 1 chart in Appendix: The Medical Hierarchy – Defining Medical Teams.)

- Try to understand why your loved one is in the hospital/ICU to begin with, digesting as much as you can about "why" the surgery, the risks, the recovery and even the worst-case scenario are important. It helps if you've asked these questions of your attending physician in advance of surgery. If you haven't, then ask for a reasonable outline from your medical lead.

- Keep handwritten and dated notes in a dedicated notebook. In that notebook, keep the following basic information and have it with you at all times:

  » A list of the patient's current medications and allergies. This is important, because medications are the hardest aspect of patient admission. Electronic records can't keep up because the patient may have added or discontinued some meds. The single source of truth about meds comes directly from the patient. It's challenging for hospitals to get the correct information, and incorrect information can obviously contribute to patient harm. Your pharmacy can help with that list.

  » Ask the primary care physician for a one-page outline of your loved one's past medical history from the patient records—a list of only the major key findings. Doctors don't have time to read a stack of medical records, but a list of key medical background is helpful: cancer, diabetes, heart failure, arthritis, asthma, etc. Your loved one may have had a particular test in another hospital in a different state. Have a hard copy of that report on hand.

» With a complex illness, like cancer treatment or an organ transplant, have a sheet of separate details and only give that to the specialists.

» List contact information of other physicians involved with your loved one's care: a gastroenterologist, primary care physician, oncologist, or any other important physicians whom you may need to be in touch with at some point.

» You can even ask for the lab reports of tests while hospitalized and keep a hard copy in your notebook in case it's needed later at a different hospital.

» In times of stress, it's only human to have trouble remembering every single thing that's been said in a complex discussion. Physicians come and go quickly, so don't be afraid to ask if you can use your phone to record a conversation or take photos. "I want to make sure I remember this so I don't ask the same questions over and over. Do you mind if I record, or take a photo?" The recordings and photos will help the doctors avoid having to repeat themselves, and they'll appreciate that. Reading the transcript of your conversation with the physician may help you form future questions more precisely. You can pass the transcribed printed pages along to the others on your family advocate team. And be respectful, of course. *Always* ask permission. This is not a "gotcha" thing. It's meant to help families. Should a particular doctor decline to be recorded, and some will, put the phone away and take your time handwriting your dated notes.

» Do speak up if something bothers you. Don't let the doctors leave the room before you've asked your questions. Take a deep breath and ask your questions in a non-confrontational way. Nobody expects families or patients to be pleasant under stress, but being hysterical or rude is not helpful in any way.

How to Open a Dialogue with Physicians

- Remember that doctors have limited time and are only going to offer so much information. They may even ask what you're most concerned about. But it's helpful if the patient speaks up, or if the advocate steps in if it's too difficult for the patient. Tell them your deepest concerns.

- First and foremost, when doctors come into the hospital room, give them a few minutes to get their bearings and assess the patient situation. After they've had a chance to digest, then ask your questions. Many times the family is scared about something that is ancillary to the important issue. So allowing time for assessment benefits everyone.

- Don't be afraid to start a dialogue. Many people don't know what to ask doctors who come in and out of the hospital room. Introduce yourself and find out who they are with a simple, "What service are you from?"

- If you want to know something, you're going to have to ask the questions. The doctor is probably thinking, "I'm going to be late for my next three patients." Just acknowledge they are busy and ask for a short amount of time, then address your thoughtful concern: "I know you're really busy. I need a minute of your time to explain this."

- Medical professionals realize that what may be common sense from a medical standpoint is not always common sense to families and patients. Just try your best to open a dialogue. There are no silly questions.

  - To get the most out of your conversation, ask one or two open-ended questions:

  "How are things going for my loved one today?"

  "Where are things going from here?"

  "Where are we now in the spectrum of my loved one's recovery? Doing perfectly well? Ahead of the curve? To be expected?"

  "What happens if … ?"

  "Doctor, I don't know what to ask. If you were in my situation right now, what would you do?"

- If you have important information about your loved one, make sure you tell everyone on the team. Don't assume that the information has been passed along. Many people think, *I've told the nurse "X", so now everyone knows.* That's not always the case.

- When and how to bring up a concern you feel is being overlooked: Dr. Speicher clarified it best. "The advocate is there at the bedside and will see much more than the primary care nurse, who is being pulled in many different directions during a busy shift. The ICU team has rounds, people are in and out, morning and afternoon. You know your loved one far better than anyone. If your intuition tells you something seems serious or isn't right, and you feel a level of certainty, bring it up first with the nurse. 90% of questions or concerns can be answered by the bedside nurse. They can flag the issue to keep watch. The nurse can bump it up and get the ball rolling with the physicians."

  If you're more concerned or not getting a response, it's good to say to the nurse, "I'm getting more concerned about this. Can you please call the doctor to check it out?"

  One of two things will happen:

  1. The white coats will educate you on why things are not adding up, and that will help you understand what's going on, or...

2. You'll provide some insight on the patient that will help the white coats in their care plan.

On the flip side, remember that when doctors are paged, they have twenty other calls just like yours. They have to triage. "Where do I go first?" The nurse will discuss with the doctor.

- Be understanding that most doctors and nurses have more work on their plates than can be humanly managed. At baseline, they are overworked and pulled in all directions. Being organized with questions and observations is a great help.

- For the advocate: It's important to get your rest. Your loved one is going to need you at full capacity when they come home. While in the ICU, medical pros are there to take care of the patient. If you have nothing left and your energy is completely spent, it's hard to do your best when the patient comes home. Yet you still have to be engaged while in the hospital. So please try to share the role with others, such as friends and family, who are willing to work as a team. As the lead advocate, organize a team schedule and figure out when it's best to be at the hospital. Sometimes it's best for family to stay overnight if the patient is having a hard time sleeping or needs comforting at night. Share information and share the time burden. Everyone benefits.

A Physician Defines a Helpful Advocate:

Dr. Speicher, our surgery fellow on Dr. D'Amico's team at the time of Rick's stay at Duke, shared great insight into how patient advocates can helpfully participate:

"Most patients need someone to help navigate minute to minute. Without an advocate, it's hard to know what motivates the patient, especially if the patient can't communicate."

"The value for doctors is in that objective third party, not of the medical team, who can take a step back and try to make sense of what's happening. The advocate consistently observes the patient for hours every day. They often recognize changes too subtle for the medical team to see immediately. Ask non-confrontational questions in order to bring attention to the issue. Speaking up about what only you know to be your loved one's baseline behavior can be helpful in giving the doctors a frame of reference."

Qualities Physicians Admire in the Best Advocates:

- One who realizes that the primary relationship is between the physician and the patient— not physician and advocate.

- The ability to develop a positive and trusting relationship with the medical team (sometimes called "providers") without acting as a "traffic cop" or going rogue. This will enable helpful communication.

- One who puts the patient in the center of attention and places their wishes and care first. Some advocates will subconsciously put their own wishes over that of the patient's, especially at the end of life, for example. Everyone understands it's terribly difficult to part with our loved ones. Those who put the selfish part of love on hold in favor of the patient's wishes are truly valuable.

- Self-centered drama diverts energy from the patient to the advocate. The best advocates try their best not to express grief as anger and aggression.

- The ability to open a positive dialogue with the doctors, including asking the right questions that may sometimes be uncomfortable.

- Someone who lends an extra perspective besides that of the patient, so the larger picture can be seen. For example, knowledge of the patient's usual baseline behavior or health can help give an important frame of reference to the medical team.

- One who knows the wishes of the patient, has an updated health care power of attorney and helps to keep priorities aligned if the patient cannot speak for themselves.

- One who does not become the patient, but rather coaches the patient if they can speak for themselves: "Do you still want to ask about...?"

- The best advocate is more than a companion. They're engaged and observant, so that when things just aren't adding up, they will speak up to the nurses or doctors without hesitation and in a non-confrontational way.

What Definitely Does Not Help the Patient, Advocate and Medical Team:

- Dr. Ofri: "Recognize that the medical teams are always overburdened, so please try to be judicious with calls and requests. It's not common but there will always be people who call every ten minutes with questions that are not urgent, or ask the same questions over and over again, or request things that are not possible to deliver. It's not common, but it only takes one or two like this to sink a doctor. I have a few patients who've figured out my personal email and send me constant messages about things that are not urgent. I appreciate the concern but it's exhausting."

- Dr. Speicher: "Being overly aggressive every minute creates a 'reputation' among the medical team that is not helpful to the advocate."

- Dr. D'Amico: "Don't go rogue or be a traffic cop. Better results come if we trust one another."

What the Nurses Want You to Know

In terms of daily care and recovery of our loved one, the bedside nurse is our greatest asset. It's not unusual for critically ill patients and their families to privately describe their bedside nurse as "sent from God, an angel sent to comfort their loved one." Yet nurses are rarely acknowledged for their great work. They mostly hear complaints. Perhaps because of this, and perhaps because of how I handled our experience with Rick's self-extubation (I'll tell you about it later), the Duke ICU nurses, as fantastic as they are, were hesitant to be interviewed for this section.

However, I was fortunate to have one exquisite Duke ICU nurse sit down with me. Her name is Bethlehem Peters. She cared for Rick quite often during his nearly eight weeks in the ICU. She is an exemplary nurse and was a wonderful person throughout Rick's ICU stay.

Pay close attention to the comments from my interview with Bethlehem. She quickly reminded me that nurses are taught to be the patient advocate. It's one of the core foundations of nursing. I had no idea until she brought it up, and that insight, in retrospect, would have been very helpful to know. Dr. D'Amico was the first to mention during his interview that the bedside nurse can answer 90% of our questions.

Although Bethlehem's comments for bedside advocates are from the Duke cardiothoracic intensive care unit perspective, you'll see her insight can apply to hospitalization in general.

Q: What concerns you most when a patient has no bedside advocate?

A: "If a patient is intubated or critical, we need a family advocate. We need an accessible advocate, even if only by phone, accessible at all times."

Q: When do you recommend an advocate get involved, or get out of the way?

A: "Research shows that family presence during stressful times is a good thing if they are emotionally stable and can stand there quietly in the background. Or, we will escort them out. Literature says it's a good thing. But if they're emotionally unstable, passing out, yelling or freaking out, a nurse will be delegated to explain what's happening. Family members are okay, but they cannot get in the way of care."

Tips for the Advocate from the Nurse's Perspective:

- Try to get a foundational understanding of what ICU care is. At Duke, the attending physician oversees the patient's overall care, and many in a surgical ICU are thrown off guard to learn their surgeon is no longer their point of contact, that the ICU nurses are now assuming that role.

- Use an organizational chart to digest the different roles of the nursing team. (See Figure 2 chart in Appendix: The Nursing Hierarchy – Defining Nursing Team Members.)

- The relationship is between the patient and nurse first. The family advocate comes second. Please don't interrupt when a nurse is working with the patient.

- Be conscious of shift changes. Find out when your hospital shift change takes place, because hospitals are different. At Duke, for example, there is a hand-off to a new nurse every twelve hours—at 7 a.m. and 7 p.m. Duke ICU nurses have two critically ill patients to care for, so they are incredibly busy during the shift change. It could be a couple of hours into their shift before nurses have a spare moment to give a status update to the family.

- Don't interrupt shift-change reports between nurses, which is given at the beginning of a new shift. This distraction can be a safety issue. It's okay sometimes to listen, but please don't interrupt. Take notes and ask your questions at the end of the hand-off.

- Each shift change is a good time to give the nurse your phone number and set specific expectations as to when you'd like to be called, night or day. Write your name and phone number in big letters on the whiteboard that is in every hospital room. Point out that information and say, "This is my phone number. Please call me at any time for these reasons: [for example] If my husband is calling for me, call me no matter what time. If my husband takes a serious downturn, please call me immediately so I can come quickly. I'm only a few minutes away."

- Ask the nurse for a preferred time for you to call them for a status update. For example, during the night shift, ask if you can call at 10 p.m. and 2 a.m. Calling halfway through the shift for an update is reasonable. But it's best to ask each nurse when to call in.

ICU Basic Etiquette Pointers:

Nurses much prefer that you ring the call bell rather than come to the nurses' station with questions. They really don't like us standing in the nurses' station.

For many reasons, including the privacy of other patients, don't stand in the hallway. Be aware of designated family areas if you need to leave the patient's hospital room.

Have a dialogue with your nurse. As I learned, "Patients and advocates listen too often and don't ask enough questions of the nurse."

No need to apologize for asking questions of a nurse. When is a good time to ask questions? Any time *except* when a nurse is directly interacting in patient care or handing off care at a shift change.

When the nurse hands off to the next shift, there is a place on their record for "events that happened today" and "plans for tomorrow." So to tie into that, it makes sense to ask these questions of each nurse at the beginning and end of the shift:

- At the beginning of the shift: "What is the plan for today?" PT? CT scan?

- At the end of the shift: "Where are we going tomorrow?"

It helps us understand the provider's linear plan and what has been accomplished. Your questions force a plan expectation. It helps to set goals and put you in synch with the nurse.

Remember to engage with your loved one who is in the hospital. Family members sometimes think they can't touch their loved one in the hospital. But normal engagement helps to ground the patient, like everyday conversation, holding hands, playing cards, watching a great sporting event on TV or listening to an audio book together.

Taking notes will help. Patients and bedside advocates who write things down tend to see the bigger picture sooner and can ask better questions.

Get involved with listening in on rounds. Listening can help you understand what's happening with the patient. Civilians have trouble understanding the language, so take notes and ask questions at the end of rounds, when the doctors have finished but are still in the room. Do not interrupt during rounds. And remember, the doctors have limited time. If you feel uncomfortable asking questions, let your nurses know and they'll ask your questions, or they'll get an answer for you. "I heard this word. Can you explain?" Nurses will advocate for you if you're the least bit intimidated to ask your questions after rounds.

Try to get a sense as to when rounds will happen, because the timing can be unpredictable. Even if you're in the room and need to get a bite to eat, ask the nurse to text you when rounds are coming so you can be back to listen in.

The Nurse's Perspective: Handling Issues of Concern:

It should go without saying, but be respectful of the nursing team from the start. Sometimes nurses are unfairly blamed for a patient's downturn, and grief in the form of rage is unloaded on them.

If there is an issue, good or bad, the charge nurse will listen to concerns and take action to be sure the best possible care is given. The charge nurse is an important role in the ICU. They can coordinate actions and be very helpful to all concerned.

For example, if you're having a great experience with a particular nurse, you can request that they be assigned to your loved one as much as possible. It's actually easier for a nurse to be in the same room repeatedly, because there are benefits to continuity of care. Or, let's say your loved one reacts well to male nurses. Ask for a male nurse to be assigned. It can be a staffing resource issue; but if staffing is available, the nursing team will do their best to get it done.

If things seem to be going wrong, hard as it might be sometimes, treat everyone with common courtesy and respect. But if the family members experience a particular nurse they don't like, for personality reasons or otherwise, there is a process to request different staffing. Advocates are encouraged to speak with the charge nurse on duty and say something like, "We've had great care in this unit; however, this particular nurse was not one who supported us in the way we needed. In the future, we'd appreciate not having this particular nurse assigned to my loved one's care."

Nurses can also request not to be assigned to a particular family or room because of the way they were treated. When a nurse becomes uncomfortable with the way a family, advocate or the patient is treating them, fatigue may set in. So, to provide the best care and prevent fatigue, a nurse can ask to be assigned elsewhere.

What Role Does Your Faith Play in Your Practice of Medicine?

I asked that question of each white coat I interviewed. Their answers were revealing.

Dr. Thomas D'Amico: "The doctor has to work with people all over the spectrum of spirituality. Some people fully believe everything is in God's hands and are at peace with that. Faith is used as a source of strength for the worst time in their life. I do not personally pray before surgery as if it would change the outcome. My physician's assistant is a deacon and does pray with patients. People always ask me at the last minute if I'm a Christian. It brings patients comfort when I say, 'Yes, I am.'"

Dr. Paul Speicher: "My faith guides how I interact with patients and how I see people as humans and that we're all in this together. I try not to project my beliefs and priorities on other people. They have the right to their own beliefs and practices. As a physician, it is not my place to try to put what I believe on anyone else. If a patient wants to pray, I'm happy to pray with them. I won't go out of my way to do it unless it is what they want. My faith guides my life, but I won't impose it on my patients."

Dr. Danielle Ofri: "I don't consciously think about spirituality. But when I'm overwhelmed and find myself slipping into a depersonalized mode, 'Oh, not *another* patient!' I try to force myself to reimagine it on a personal level. 'What if that patient were my father, or my grandmother, or my child?' How would I want their doctor to think about them, to treat them? That's what I lean on."

"I'm not especially religious, although my father was. Judaism was the most important pillar in his life and he chanted the weekly Torah portion aloud for his synagogue every week for decades. There is a saying in the Talmud, 'If you save one life it's like you save the world.' I lean on that a lot. It's easy to feel defeated because the system is so overwhelming. But if you can move the needle one degree for one patient, it's like you've saved the world for that person. For the patient who lost their reading glasses after being transferred from one hospital room to another … if you can find those glasses, then you've changed their world, even if it's just a little bit."

"There is so much to do that you can get completely over-whelmed by it all. I try to remind myself that I need to do one thing for one person to make a difference whether it's making that one extra phone call, or tracking down the right case worker, or sorting out the one mixed-up prescription."

"That's on a good day. On my worst days, I'm sobbing in my office."

Bethlehem Peters, RN, BSN: "I pray every day, 'Give me the words to speak to patients and their families and strength to endure.' I pray to be selfless. It's important for me to leverage my faith so my patients can see I serve them and I serve through God."

Through the Advocate's Eyes

THE FIRST FEW DAYS

I learned my very first lessons within 24 hours of Rick's early morning surgery, April 16, 2018.

He was in the surgical ICU by midday. The 7th floor ICU room had large windows to let in the sun, along with a view of the outside world. A nurse attended to Rick, who was waking from an esophagectomy, a complicated surgery. He had a tube the size of a small garden hose in his lower right side draining fluids, and thankfully he was full of meds, so he was not in any pain. Kelly, Stephen and I were there surrounding Rick, who eventually stood up with the help of his nurses and took a seat in the large recliner that seems to be in every hospital room, propped up, facing the sunny window.

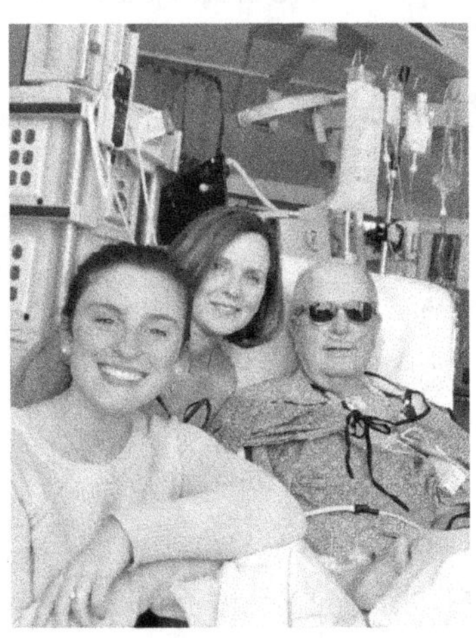

Rick with Kelly and Kim in ICU

Dr. Sara Najmeh, a surgery fellow at the time, was the first of Dr. D'Amico's team to come by Rick's ICU room on April 16, 2018. She took time to literally draw out a simplified description of the surgery for us on a white board.

Dr. Sara, as she asked us to call her, had a lovely precision in her physical movement and in her conversation. Although educated in Canada, Dr. Sara originally came from Syria, where her parents still lived. We all agreed she was beautiful and had an elegant way of redirecting a conversation to stay on track. She got Rick's sense of humor right away, and we loved how Rick enjoyed talking to Dr. Sara. Whether offering to "fact check" the Fox News show she caught on his TV, or listening to his heart's desire to go home, have a vodka martini and enjoy life again, she made Rick feel like he was her only patient, even though she had a million other things to do.

Several weeks later, Dr. Sara had rotated away from Rick's care, but she'd stop by occasionally to look in on him. Rick was still in the ICU, intubated on a ventilator, and he seemed totally unconscious to us whenever she came by.

On one of those occasions she'd been up all night participating in heart transplant surgery. She was visibly weary, but she came to Rick's bedside anyway. She took his hand, gazed at him for several minutes without speaking, and then quietly offered encouraging words to us. To this day, we still remember her kindness and hope she knows how much it meant to us.

When he was conscious, Rick would banter with and tease the nurses who came in and out of his ICU room. They were friendly and laughed a bit with us. "This is going to be fine," I thought. "Wonderful nurses, positive and attentive."

We had been told by Dr. D'Amico in the pre-op clinic that it was unlikely Rick would experience terrible pain. Some discomfort, yes, but the "pain-management team" knew how to handle it. "We've seen everything," he said, "and we can manage the pain." We enjoyed the afternoon of April 16 with Rick, and his spirits were good.

I left him that evening to go back to the hotel a few minutes away to get a night's rest. When Kelly and I returned the next morning, April 17, we found that Rick could barely breathe, he was in so much pain. My strong husband—the one from whom in thirty-four years I'd rarely heard even a passing comment about pain, through injuries and three other surgeries—had been in excruciating pain during the night. He told me he'd been crying out for me, but I didn't come. I'd never heard a comment like that from my husband. As you can imagine, Kelly and I were heartbroken.

Rick's pain meds had been all but stopped the night before because of his blood pressure and other concerns. During rounds that day I brought up the pain issues to Dr. D'Amico while Dr. Sara listened. He kind of dismissed it, saying, "Well, people react differently to pain." He was understandably more focused on attending to Rick's overall status. I didn't know what to make of Dr. D'Amico's comment, but Rick's pain was under control at the moment, so we moved on.

"Pain is subjective. We really don't know what another person feels," the nurses kept telling me. Right. But I know my husband better than anyone else on Earth, and I'd never seen him react like this to pain. (Months later, while interviewing Dr. D'Amico, he said, "The family's interpretation of pain is always inaccurate.")

Regardless of what anyone else had to say, it was clear to us: We had to watch over Rick's pain management.

I was completely out of my element, though, and I needed qualified help to make sure Rick's pain was managed in the future. I called my friend Darlene, a nurse manager in a large South Carolina hospital. She talked me through it from the nurse's perspective. I had no org chart, so she gave me a verbal "chain of command" for the ICU, and she coached me on how to effectively speak about pain to the bedside nurses, nurse management team, and physicians. She was emphatic that I had "every right to call the lead physician if you feel pain is not being managed well."

While I worked on insurance issues during that afternoon, Kelly watched over her dad in his ICU room. Rick wasn't in as much pain by then but was still shaken from that previous night. He was apprehensive, a different person. She observed a technician in his room who she felt was "too rough" while doing tests and seemed to mock his pain.

Concerned, Kelly went out in the hallway to look for his nurse. She was met by a familiar face, Bethlehem, who asked if she could help. Kelly voiced her concern about the technician, and without hesitation, Bethlehem walked into Rick's room to observe. Her physical presence alone was comforting. From then on, the nurses would stop in and stand at Rick's bedside when technicians came in and out to work on him—observing, helping, and there for us. It made all the difference in Rick's care, and it was our first wave of sheer gratitude for them. *May God bless the nurses.*

The night shift change brought us a new nurse to care for Rick, and she was a godsend. She patiently listened to my concerns from the previous night. "What should be done so this pain episode doesn't happen again?" I asked her.

She didn't just hear me, she actually took the time to make eye contact. "On my watch, he will not be in pain, to the very best of my ability. I promise. And I will call you if necessary." Exactly what I needed to hear.

That accomplished, I kept right on following my friend Darlene's coaching instructions. One by one, I asked to speak with each person on the ICU team who would be taking care of Rick that night—the bedside nurse, then the charge nurse (in the presence of the bedside nurse), then the intensivist, who sent a young male resident to speak to me. Still in front of the bedside nurse, I asked the resident, "Who was responsible for stopping my husband's pain meds last night?"

"I was," he replied.

"Where was the pain-management team I was told would be available?"

"On the phone with me," he said.

"My husband's pain management didn't work very well," I told him. "I plan to call Dr. D'Amico myself this evening if we feel his pain isn't well managed."

I'd been coached to ask the bedside nurse if she had all the orders necessary for pain, which I did in front of the resident. The resident stepped away to discuss something with the nurse, maybe for my benefit, already knowing how things would go. Even so, I'm still grateful, because it really was all I could do.

Then the resident turned back to me and said, "You're his advocate. I get it."

I'd never thought about, let alone used the word "advocate", before. I simply said, "Yes well, I hope you'll do your best to see to it that he is not in pain."

He promised to do his "very best." It was beginning to sound like a refrain.

I share this conversation because that was the day I realized we couldn't leave Rick alone in the hospital ever again. We had to step it up and get organized.

Here are the rookie mistakes I made and some things I learned:

- Until my friend Darlene coached me, I was clueless about the chain of command in the ICU; and not everyone is fortunate enough to have a coach like I did. Now *you've* got an org chart as a starting reference.

- I didn't leave my name and phone number on the white board, nor did I ask to have it marked in their records with clear, specific instructions to call me if Rick should start going downhill. If I had, a nurse would have called me. My hotel was literally five minutes away, and I could have been there for him. Lesson learned.

- On that first night (and every night), staying until the 7 p.m. shift change is important. Once the nurses finished handing off by giving "report," I should have introduced myself to the new night nurse. "I'm Mrs. Norris. Thank you for taking care of my husband. I'm going back to my hotel, but is it okay to call you at 10 p.m. and 2 a.m. to ask about his status?" That simple act would have enabled me to be there for Rick when he was in so much pain. And remember, the shift change is the best time to set specific instructions on where and when you'd liked to be contacted. The white board on the wall of each and every hospital room is your and your loved one's caregiver's friend.

- When speaking to the nurses by phone for a status update, be prepared with one or two straightforward questions, such as:

  "Is he able to sleep? If not, what is the plan?"

  "Is he in pain? If so, what is the plan?"

  "Is there a downturn?"

- It's important to know how the pain-management team works and have their contact information if available. If I'd been there witnessing my husband's pain, I'd have every right to ask the nurse to call someone to manage it.

- It only took one night in the ICU to learn to be grateful for good bedside nurses. Rick was in the ICU for almost two months, and during that time we tried to find ways to show our appreciation for all the nurses on shift. Believe me, I was a difficult advocate at times, so showing some gratitude was in order. I learned that individual gifts cannot be given to nurses—the entire shift has to receive the gift. So I catered lunch for the entire day shift, and coffee and food for the entire night shift during one particular 24-hour span. We asked what the nurses liked to eat, and then ordered good sandwiches, salads and dessert from a local restaurant. A small gesture, really: They deserve so much more.

- Ask your nurse for help. Kelly and I were both new at this and didn't know that the nurses see themselves as patient advocates. When we talked to the nurses working in the room next to ours, they made time to help us.

Challenging the Doctor

There may be a time when things get very stressful, and an outburst erupts between the advocate and the physicians. It happened to me, and I'm including this story because it illustrates how everyone involved benefits when there is trust between physician, patient and advocate. Sometimes trust has to be reinforced by actions.

Around May 6, Rick had acute respiratory failure. It was serious enough that we were called into the ICU that Sunday morning by the surgery fellow on duty. Rick was critically ill and was intubated on a ventilator. The ventilator was not helping because fluid had accumulated between the lungs and the chest wall, making it impossible for him to breathe. He needed a procedure to drain the fluid. Stephen led Kelly and me in prayer as we stood next to Rick's bed in the ICU.

Then Stephen, Kelly, the surgery fellow on Dr. D'Amico's team, the ICU bedside nurse and I all crowded into an elevator around Rick's hospital bed and the ventilator on the way to the radiology department for the procedure. The fellow was a tiny young woman, and we'd had one short conversation early on when Rick was rushed back to the ICU for a few stressful days before recovering under her watch.

Now, in the elevator, with no room to spare, I stood next to the surgeon, who turned to me and said, "Remember when you asked me to let you know when things are seriously critical? Well, if this procedure doesn't help your husband, there is only one other option:

an ECMO. It's a procedure to bypass the lungs and oxygenate the blood. Not all hospitals have this capability, but we do. If we have to go with that option, it can only be done for a short time. Then there will be no further options."

It was a surreal moment. All I could say was, "Well, then ... I guess my husband's life is in your hands."

She discreetly took my left hand and said quietly, "I'll do my very best."

We arrived at the X-ray department and parted ways with the white coats. The waiting areas were completely empty, and we were directed to a small room across the hall. I stepped around the corner to another deserted waiting room and called Rick's lifelong friends Tom and Joy Jackson to let them know, and I prayed again for mercy.

The doctors drained about a liter of fluid, I was told. Rick was again given a chance to recover and was able to stay on the ventilator instead of needing the ECMO option.

We were at his bedside throughout the days following that difficult Sunday. Rick was still on the ventilator and looked completely unconscious. I would turn my back to Rick's bed and stand facing out of his window to cry in case he could somehow hear me. The nurse brought tissues, asking "Do you need anything?" and then giving me privacy.

The nurses began recommending a tracheostomy for Rick instead of being intubated on a ventilator. This procedure entails making an opening in the neck to insert a tube into the windpipe, allowing air into the lungs

I had a bad feeling about the tracheostomy, but the nurses lobbied for it. They pressed to speak to Dr. D'Amico on our behalf, one nurse calling it "inhumane" to keep Rick intubated for so long. Yet, the surgery fellow said that there were risks to a tracheostomy. It could become permanent, and it could cause damage that could, in turn, cause more suffering. Since things seemed to be going wrong for Rick, that scared me.

To this point, we'd rarely seen Dr. D'Amico himself. Instead, there had been plenty of swirling physicians, residents, nurses, specialists we didn't know, all sorts of people in and out, mostly not speaking to us. I didn't do very well with asking questions of them.

One afternoon, in came Dr. D'Amico and three others, presumably his students. One of them was Dr. Paul Speicher, the surgery fellow who would turn out to be so important to us.

They entered the room and gathered around the foot of Rick's bed. I stood and said nothing. They talked about things I didn't understand and began discussing a tracheostomy for Rick. Their conversation seemed cold and dismissive of the suffering Rick was enduring. I was heartbroken and sorrowful but hiding it well, I thought.

When Dr. D'Amico completed his session he turned to me and asked, "How are you doing?"

My grief welled up. "How am I doing? I'm pissed off. That's how I'm doing." I stood next to Rick and told Dr. D'Amico in front of his students that if we'd known how brutal this surgery would be, we probably would have opted out. The surgery was supposed to have given us more time together, I told him, not accelerate and intensify his suffering. "I didn't know the right questions to ask you. I wish I had."

Dr. D'Amico, a gifted, revered surgeon by all accounts, shot back, "Well, if you *had* asked, I would have told you this surgery is your husband's best chance to survive."

"Well, then, why is my husband doing so badly? Why is he suffering so much? Instead of talking about a trach, how about having someone find out why he keeps getting pneumonia?"

The students, who I'm pretty sure weren't expecting this kind of conversation, were all looking straight ahead at the wall, except Dr. Speicher, who looked at me with a wide-open expression, listening intently. I motioned toward them and said to Dr. D'Amico, "I'm grateful to be here at Duke, but it's not their job to take care of my husband. You are responsible, and I want to know why he is suffering so much."

Dr. D'Amico started to respond, but I put my hand up. "Just talk to me when you find out what's wrong with my husband."

To his credit, Dr. D'Amico led his students out of the room without saying another word.

Hours later I was told Dr. D'Amico was going to do a procedure the next morning to see what was going on. For all I knew, that procedure had already been planned well before my outburst. If so, nobody told me about it. But then, I hadn't asked the question, either.

Regardless, the following day, around noon, I was in the 7 West ICU waiting room wolfing down sushi from a plastic cafeteria container. Finally, the procedure over, Dr. D'Amico came out alone, found me and sat down. He flipped over a used piece of paper, drew a picture and described the procedure he'd done.

Rick, it turned out, had a leak in his reconstructed esophagus and another tear in his windpipe (as I understood it). The digestive fluids were going into Rick's lungs, causing respiratory problems. Dr. D'Amico placed a stent in the esophagus to contain the fluids and give the tears enough time to heal.

"I'm not going to do the tracheostomy. We're going to give him time to heal as he is."

I exhaled for the first time in what felt like weeks. "Thank you, Dr. D'Amico. That's all I ever wanted to know."

That day restored my faith in him. In spite of his insanely busy schedule, he'd taken the time to personally do the procedure and then provide the information that meant so much. He came alone and talked with me one-on-one. I truly appreciated that. For us rookies, sometimes all it takes is action from that one important individual to restore our trust and make us better advocates for our loved ones.

Later, during my interviews with both Dr. D'Amico and Dr. Speicher, I asked, "What does it feel like to be challenged by a family advocate?" Here are their replies:

Dr. D'Amico told me, "If the family doesn't feel like they've been given enough information, then the doctor deserves it. We hope it doesn't get to that point with a good relationship. In times of stress, even when it feels like a personal attack, the doctors can't get defensive. If you have questions as an advocate, 90% of them can be answered by someone who is not the main attending doctor. The bedside nurse is the first line of questions. If they can't answer and you need a doctor, ask the nurse when one will be available."

Dr. Speicher went further and explained his full-force listening that day as I choked out my grief and fear. "When I first came into your room, I got the impression you didn't really understand how complex Rick's operation was. It's hard to explain, especially when things aren't going well. For those early in training it's uncomfortable, but I'm not uncomfortable at this time. In those situations it's about you, the advocate, not the patient. We're doing all we can scientifically for the patient, but you don't know that. So you're angry and frustrated and scared. You've never been here before, so you don't care about making a doctor feel uncomfortable. When I walk into that situation it's mostly about listening to you and understanding what you're scared about. Where are you going with that? Sometimes people just want to know if their loved one is going to survive, but it hurts too much to ask that directly. Or they want to know when their loved one is coming home but don't know how to ask the question. We want to know exactly what we're talking about … get on the same page."

He helpfully concluded, "When the advocate starts out defensive and angry before trying to understand the bigger picture, it hurts the dialogue, and everyone benefits from a good dialogue. Medicine is complicated, and it's sometimes difficult to explain in two sentences that what may seem harmful really is not. It's harder for the doctor to explain what's going on if the advocate has already decided I'm an idiot or evil or disengaged."

Lessons learned

- I learned that there can be no peace without trust in something or someone—whether a doctor, the nurses, a higher spiritual power or the medical team as a community. The positive effects are going to be felt by all concerned if there is trust—hopefully, layers upon layers of trust. That trust for me is built on actions by the individual and good communication. The loss of trust, as I experienced, is completely detrimental to good advocacy, good relationships and good health.

- Doctors I interviewed told me that plenty of patients don't want to know the details. They leave it completely in the hands of their medical team. But for those of us who need to understand, especially when a critically ill loved one cannot speak for themselves or are intubated on a ventilator, we must ask the hard questions. The doctors and nurses do not have time to offer up too much information, nor did I experience that they commonly have time to ask about our fears. It's going to be better for everyone if the advocate focuses on asking the right questions.

- Instead of letting my fear and grief build up, it would have been more productive to reach out to the bedside nurses. It would have been helpful if someone had let me know the deeper role of the ICU nurse as patient advocate in advance of terribly stressful events. Now you know.

- This is a good time to mention that I felt better when I gave myself a break once in a while. Breaks as simple as taking a 20-minute walk, or sitting down to lunch in a cafe, or taking a few minutes to chat with a stranger at the coffee station on the ICU floor. Even if it felt like I was pretending all was well, the smallest break seemed to build up a tiny reserve of gratitude and optimism.

- Once your question is cleared by the nurse, do speak up to the attending physician when you have the chance (without interrupting rounds). Non-confrontational is always best. The physicians will engage and help.

SELF-EXTUBATION

The longer the stay in any hospital, the higher the likelihood that something will go wrong. Medical professionals and advocates are doing their best, but we are all imperfect human beings, and bad things happen, in spite of our best efforts—especially, it seems, at night.

This is the story of one such event that happened to Rick that put us at odds with the medical professionals. It's a good teaching moment for everyone.

While in the cardiothoracic surgical ICU at Duke, Rick had been on a ventilator for almost two weeks, recovering from acute respiratory failure as I described earlier.

The nurses counseled me over the weeks that, because the ventilator was extremely uncomfortable for Rick, the sedatives had to be "titrated." This means that they had to be continually measured and balanced, to keep him somewhat conscious yet well sedated to mitigate his discomfort. Otherwise he would become agitated and try to pull out the ventilator tube, also known as self-extubation.

He was to lay back in his bed at a thirty-degree angle that made it a bit easier for him to reach his respirator tube. The tube has a cuff or balloon at the end, and once it's placed in the windpipe (trachea) the balloon is inflated. So you can imagine how uncomfortable it might be to pull out an inflated object from your windpipe.

For his protection, Rick's hands needed to be restrained when left alone in the room, even momentarily. The bedside nurses were almost apologetic about the soft restraints, calling it a necessary precaution. It was very important, I was told time and again, that he not pull out the ventilator tube.

The stent Dr. D'Amico placed in Rick's esophagus on May 11, 2018, was working. His severe respiratory issues had been successfully relieved, and Rick was doing well enough to be freed. Dr. D'Amico ordered that his ventilator be removed on Friday, May 18. We were thrilled.

The night before, on May 17, 2018, Kelly and I waited in Rick's room for the nurse shift change. It was a very busy night, the charge nurse told us, and it did seem chaotic in the cardiothoracic surgical ICU. Kelly and I stood by Rick's bed. He seemed unconscious. One of our favorite nurses was coming on duty that evening … but then, a last-minute change. That nurse was assigned elsewhere, and a different nurse was assigned to Rick instead.

Rick had been in the ICU for about a month, but we'd never seen this particular nurse before. After we introduced ourselves, I pointed out my contact information on the white board in Rick's room and asked to be called should anything happen during the night.

Then we added that we'd learned his soft restraints were necessary when left alone and hoped the focus would be on making sure Rick was comfortable throughout the night, with well-balanced sedatives that would let him have a night's rest.

The nurse responded with a comment that seemed cavalier, a bit too casual: "Yeah, I'll mess around with it." It was unlike anything said by any of the other nurses we'd experienced there. I dismissed it, as things were very busy, and we needed to get out of the way. But as we walked out of the ICU, I said to Kelly, "I don't have a good feeling about the night nurse."

On the 30-minute drive home, I was still unsettled. Something didn't seem right, and I became emotional when we arrived at our apartment in Raleigh. I attributed it to exhaustion.

Late that night, we learned that this particular night nurse was not as diligent as he should have been. Rick's medication was apparently not well balanced after all, and he was very uncomfortable. The nurse left his station, as he himself told me, to use the bathroom (perfectly understandable) but did not restrain Rick's hands. With no one apparently monitoring him, Rick pulled out the ventilator tube, inflated cuff and all.

Because the stent in his esophagus was helping his recovery from his severe respiratory issues, my immediate fear was that pulling out the breathing tube could have damaged his esophagus or his windpipe, creating yet another setback to his recovery and heaping on more suffering. Would he die because of this?

Further, the nurse did not call me as requested. Perhaps he just didn't have time. I only found out because of my nightly routine of calling the nurse on duty at around 10 p.m. and 2 a.m. When the nurse answered my call that night and told me what had happened, I was completely shocked. My husband had endured weeks on a ventilator to heal from fluids leading from his esophagus to his lungs, which caused pneumonia. He was scheduled to be taken off the ventilator within hours. He was getting better. Now he may have harmed himself, and his recovery may have been set back again. More punishment to his frail body.

I couldn't contain myself. I growled through the phone at the nurse, "What the hell are you doing leaving my husband alone without restraining his hands?" He answered that restraints were not "required," although the other nurses had stressed their importance. I accused the night nurse of negligence and commanded, "Don't go near my husband! Stay out of his room!" Then I demanded to speak with the charge nurse, who quickly took the phone. The charge nurse told me to stop shouting, instantly began defending the night nurse and seemed unconcerned about Rick, which angered me even further.

"How about you concentrate on not killing my husband?!" I thundered into the phone.

I asked to speak to the intensivist (the ICU doctor on duty). She took the phone and, again, started out by protecting the nurse. "We really don't know what happened."

I shot back, "I'm not stupid and neither are you. The medication was not titrated properly, and my husband was left alone with no restraints, so he pulled out the ventilator tube. I do not give my permission for you to put that tube back into my husband. *Do not* put that tube back in unless you speak to Dr. D'Amico or his fellow on duty."

To which the intensivist, voice dripping with condescension, informed me that she would do what she felt was necessary and didn't need my permission or the surgeon's.

I was enraged. "You *better not* put that tube back in my husband unless you get Dr. D'Amico's permission!"

She replied, "You're threatening me." Then, *click*, she hung up on me.

Honestly, if I could have reached through the phone and grabbed that doctor by the throat, I would have.

Hearing all this, my daughter Kelly got out of bed. It was around 1 a.m. She took charge and directed me to "get a grip." "You're too angry to advocate properly," she said. "We show up when things are not going well, so I'm going to be with Dad."

She left and drove the thirty minutes to Duke Hospital in the middle of the night to sit by her father's bedside and protect him from any further neglect. Kelly proved to be a fierce advocate and protector of her father throughout his hospitalization... day or night.

When Kelly arrived at the ICU on the 7th floor of the Duke Medical Pavilion, the security desk had already alerted them that someone was coming up. Although the ICU receptionist knew us and would typically buzz us right in, that night Kelly was asked to wait for an escort. Two people came to meet her: the charge nurse and another person. They introduced themselves to Kelly, and in their next breath assured her that the nurse did nothing wrong. Kelly let them know that she was more concerned about her dad right now. They would talk about the nurse later, at a time of her choosing, but *not now.*

Kelly may have looked like a little 15-year-old in her sweats, but she was calm and focused and fully in charge of her emotions—a surprising force to be reckoned with. She remembers turning the corner to her dad's room to find every eye on her as she walked past the main nurses' station where the intensivist stood, and she noticed that everyone stopped talking as she walked by. We were not very popular at the moment.

She let out a huge sigh of relief when she arrived in Rick's room and was greeted by Brianna. Brianna had been Rick's nurse a few times, and she was a trusted and calming presence. She was also the only one who didn't start off by saying that the other nurse did nothing wrong. Instead, she was focused on taking care of Rick and letting Kelly know that her father was doing well.

Rick was taking deep breaths, sitting up and looking around. He seemed totally conscious and was talking somewhat normally for someone who'd been on a ventilator for two weeks. Kelly pulled the recliner next to his bed, settled in with her blanket and pillow and said to her dad, "Why did you pull out your breathing tube?"

"Why not?" was the answer.

"Don't ever do that again! It's dangerous!" his daughter and advocate scolded.

Dr. D'Amico came by later that morning, at around 5:30 a.m., and assured Kelly that her father was doing fine and that self-extubation was "not uncommon"—every doctor's favorite phrase.

The next day I came to the ICU to relieve Kelly. The new charge nurse came to speak with me and asked if I wanted to meet with management. "I'm too exhausted and not myself," I told her. "I'm not thinking clearly. If we think it's necessary, we'll address it with management at a later time when my husband is better."

Rick lasted a week breathing on his own. Then, on another night of a different day, he was given sleep medication, which apparently impacted his ability to clear his air way of mucous. He was put back on the ventilator for another week. Being on a ventilator meant he had no muscle activity for weeks, just laid in bed in an altered state of consciousness. We feared he'd have a slower recovery once he was discharged from the hospital or that he wouldn't overcome the delirium.

INFORMATION ABOUT THE RISK OF SELF-EXTUBATION

A quick search for studies on self-extubation proved enlightening. One such study – "Self-extubation in ICU patients", October 15, 2014, The Southwest Respiratory and Critical Care Chronicles—taught me that Rick was a likely candidate. He was a surgical patient older than sixty-five. He had prolonged immobility because he'd been on a ventilator for over a week already and was in the ICU for about a month, and he had delirium.

The incidence of self-extubation is higher during the night shift, and especially during shift changes when patients are less monitored. Moreover, there is a higher likelihood of self-extubation among patients who are hours away from a planned extubation. Rick was scheduled to be extubated the next day.

The studies showed that a less experienced nurse caring for a patient means a higher risk of self-extubation. The particular nurse in my husband's care told me himself that he did not restrain my husband's hands when he left Rick alone because "it is not required." Yet every other nurse went out of their way to explain why they reluctantly restrained his hands for a short time if they were busy with another patient, even when I was in the room.

Further, the information noted, it is critical to balance sedation properly to control agitation, which is another reason for unplanned self-extubation by patients. The study suggested the importance of at least one nurse monitoring patients with these attributes at all times. In the moment, we felt ours was one case of negligence by one particular nurse, but it was actually a combination of things that caused the self-extubation.

If I had only known how at risk Rick was for this, I would have stayed with him overnight. My outrage was partially fueled by my own guilt for not being there for him, and partially by my expecting *absolute perfection* from the nurses and doctors. Neither one was rational.

> ### LESSONS LEARNED
>
> - It is never, *ever* appropriate to verbally threaten a medical professional, under any circumstances, *especially* the very physicians and nurses who are caring for your critically ill loved one. Shameful lack of self-control on my part resulted in completely unproductive behavior—a terrible advocacy strategy.
>
> - My first reaction was to blame the nurse, accuse him of negligence and use the words "*kill my husband!*" In this litigious climate, no wonder the ICU team's first response was to protect the nurse. And their reaction only fueled further outrage on our part, because it seemed as if their top priority was to cover for the nurse, rather than to focus on Rick's care. Had the night nurse, or any one of the subsequent medical professionals I talked to, started out by letting me know that my husband was doing just fine and explained that self-extubation is fairly common, it would have without a doubt defused my fearful outburst. Why the contentious start? Maybe because that particular night nurse was not experienced in handling such things.
>
> - Dr. Speicher later clarified for me that self-extubation is not that uncommon. However, it is most certainly a potentially life-threatening event when it happens—someone absolutely needs to be at the bedside immediately assessing the patient. Fortunately, in the cardiothoracic intensive care unit at Duke, there

is always at least one 24/7 intensivist in-house, all of whom happen to be anesthesiologists by training and best suited to assess whether the breathing tube needs to go back in or not. Although the surgical team needs to know when it happens, the surgeon or fellow does not typically rush in. The intensivist who is already there would make the decision as to whether or not to put the tube back in and will actually do it if needed. As long as such an event is responded to promptly, bad outcomes are typically avoided. So, the intensivist had it covered that night, but we, the family, did not know it. I certainly had no idea that the intensivist was the best equipped to care for Rick's self-extubation event. Now *you* know.

- As for the conversation with the intensivist, perhaps it was an opportunity for this well-educated physician-in-charge to diffuse matters with just a little tiny touch of compassion, something like, "Your husband is okay. He did take out the ventilator tube, but he is okay. We've got him. It's probably shocking to you, but this isn't uncommon, and I'll tell you why when things calm down. I've already let Dr. D'Amico's team know. We'll have your husband talk with you in a little while if you'd like. He's okay. A new nurse is going to look after him as you requested." Any one of those comments would have stopped me in my tracks, and I probably would have dissolved into tears rather than rage.

- The intensivist was absolutely correct: She *was* in charge and didn't need my permission or direction. But the conversation, with a touch of kindness, could have ended on a much more positive note than hanging up on the terrified wife of her critically ill patient. To this day, that event is remembered by family members as one of the most negative and brutal experiences of Rick's life—"not that uncommon" or not. The ripple effect of negativity went from the patient and family to nurses, nurse management, physicians and the universe at large as we continued to talk about it. This example is one from which we can all learn to do better. There has got to be a kinder, more reasonable way.

- It would have been a great help if someone had taken a moment to share information and explain the bigger picture to us in the beginning of our experience with the ventilator. Perhaps touching on self-extubation is called for, since it's "not that uncommon." The nurses tried by talking about the soft restraints on Rick's hands. But they don't have time to educate the bedside advocate on everything, and we couldn't see the full picture. Sharing information would have been more productive for everyone, saving time and energy.

- When I sensed that the night nurse in question was a bit too casual with his "yeah, I'll mess around with it" comment, and even felt as I walked away from my husband's room that night that something wasn't right, I didn't speak up. I doubted my intuition and didn't trust that pit-of-the-stomach feeling. That was a mistake on my part.

When Everyday ICU Care Seems Like It's Not Going Well

The nursing care Rick received during his yearlong illness, especially while at Duke University, was excellent. In my experience, the Duke nurses were complete professionals, hardworking, compassionate, smart, perhaps under-appreciated, and doing the physical labor and dirty work of bedside care with strength, humor and kindness.

But nurses are indeed human, and sometimes things can be concerning for patients and families. This story is to share how well the nurse management reacted to our concerns, based on the coaching I received from my friend, herself a nurse manager at a different hospital.

Rick had been in the ICU for about six weeks after the self-extubation. He was struggling with delirium and respiratory issues, and was very weak. He had developed a bed sore that was painful, and he hadn't slept in weeks.

Each ICU nurse had two patients. Our particular nurse on duty was focused on her other patient next door, who was also very ill. I was trying to have Rick moved from his bed to a recliner or wheelchair so he could look out the window, or be brought out in the windowed hallway so he could have a change of scenery, light and fresh air, since I had been told this would help him get better and help with the delirium. He'd been in the ICU a very long time, and we were focused on trying to help him get well enough to move to the step-down unit. From there he could be discharged to a rehab hospital, and then home.

Rick began to be passed over a bit in the care process that day. Soiled bed linens were not removed from the room hamper.

Waiting for three hours to be taken out for sunlight and air, he'd finally fall into much-needed sleep but couldn't be moved when busy nurses were available to accompany him on a field trip. Or the physical therapist would come while he was having a test and wouldn't return until the next day or two, leaving him without the benefit of PT for several days. An accumulation of things like that happened all day long.

Finally the nurse, toward the end of her shift, informed me, "Your husband is not as ill as the patient next door, so you'll have to wait." Also "not uncommon," I learned.

I waited until the 7 p.m. shift change to meet the new nurse, feeling frustrated and uneasy about his care all day and troubled about how his night would go. Bad things happen at night.

The night nurse was someone we already knew was wonderful. She was busy giving report. I let her know I was going home but would call her later. On the drive home from Durham to Raleigh I worried that Rick might fall under the radar and have another setback. He'd already been through so much.

Around 9 p.m. I called the night nurse, and we had this conversation:

"I'm so grateful that you're taking care of my husband tonight, and for all the nursing care over the past weeks," I said. "But I observed some things all day today that have me very concerned."

She asked me what happened, and I explained.

"Here's what you should do ..." she told me, and she gave me the name and contact information of the night charge nurse. "Call her. She'll help you."

We'd had the self-intubation disaster weeks before, and I wanted to handle this in a more constructive way. So when I spoke to the charge nurse, I started calmly with, "My husband is Richard Norris. His nurse this evening suggested I call you about some concerns."

To her credit, the charge nurse told me to speak freely and tell her specifically what had happened.

Then, careful with my tone of voice, based on what I'd learned weeks ago, I summarized my concern with specific examples.

- "My husband has a painful bed sore on his tailbone that seems to have gotten worse. I don't think the nurse had time to look at it all day. Can someone please help him?"

- "I've been told by his physicians and the nurses that in order to help overcome delirium, my husband needs sunlight and air, and needs to get out of bed. But I observed that he missed not only his PT sessions again today but also his chance for physical activity outside the ICU."

- "The nurse said that my husband was not as sick as her other patient, and he'd have to wait for her to help move him from his bed to his wheelchair. We waited for three hours, and by that time he was too tired to be moved. I'm worried that he won't get the air and light to help him get over the delirium he's had for several weeks now."

- "The soiled bed linens were not removed from his hamper. I asked one of the nursing assistants to take them away, or I would have done it myself. I was concerned he could not have been kept clean had I not been there today."

After hearing me out, the charge nurse told me the examples were all basic nursing, and she would take care of it. She then asked me if there were any nurses that I did not want to take care of my husband. I gave her two names.

The very next morning, orders had been written for the following:

- A wound care specialist to come take care of Rick's bed sore. (I had no idea there was even such a thing as a "wound specialist." I learned they were somewhere on the floor, and all I had to do was make a request. I didn't even know enough to ask.)

- Rick to be taken out of his ICU room for air and sunlight. I didn't have to constantly ask.

Lessons learned

- Request a "wound specialist" to help your loved one with any wound, including painful bed sores.

- Since my concerns were described by examples, the charge nurse was quick to help. Having observations written down helps to clearly articulate them.

- I tried to be honest about my observations and concerns, but *not accusatory*. I'd already learned that we don't see the full picture in terms of what is going on in a hospital unit. Everyone really is trying their best.

Physical Therapy

Mobility, I learned from physicians, nurses and physical therapists, is critical to just about anyone's recovery. Moving around, getting up and walking as soon as possible, was very important to Rick's recovery, from the surgery and from the delirium.

Ken, the awesome physical therapist, came to the ICU to see Rick. Here's where I'll pass along a comment made by Dr. Speicher, *"Ken is probably personally responsible for saving at least as many lives as any doctor or nurse."* That's how important physical therapy is.

Ken talked with me and went out of his way to help Rick with PT sessions so he could get back on his feet. I learned that the physical therapists have lots of stops scheduled throughout the day, and if a patient is asleep or not in the room, they move on to the next patient. They will often run out of time to double back, so a patient can easily miss a session. That means going without physical therapy for several days if a weekend is involved.

Toward the end of Rick's nearly 11-week stay in Duke Hospital, PT continuity became an issue. He would miss his appointments, and that impacted his ability to achieve certain physical guidelines in order to be accepted into a good inpatient rehabilitation hospital.

Lessons learned

- Ask the physical therapists what the plan is, and then follow the plan. In our case, the PT pros counseled that there was a delicate balance between encouraging the therapy and rushing it to the detriment of Rick's recovery.

- Physical therapy was key to recovery. My thanks to the Duke Hospital physical therapy team for helping my husband qualify to be accepted into an excellent inpatient rehabilitation hospital near our home in Bluffton, South Carolina. It made a huge difference in his recovery and allowed him to return home to enjoy himself for a few good months. It was a hard-won pleasure to have Rick home and for us to walk around our neighborhood together, especially his victory walk down to his beloved dock on the May River.

CHAPTER SIX

ICU Delirium

By April 23, 2018, Rick's medical records noted "disrupted sleep cycle." Four days later, he was not himself. I'd never heard of "ICU delirium" or any other kind of delirium brought on by hospitalization.

Dr. Dwayne Gard told me patients more prone to delirium tend to be older, on multiple medications, including new ones such as narcotics and pain meds they're not used to. Some of them, he said, have underlying dementia already.

Please take delirium seriously, especially if it persists for weeks. In Rick's case, it lasted for two months.

When Rick's delirium was finally discussed at my request, I was given the typical response that it's "not uncommon." Did that mean it was common? Why had nobody mentioned anything about it? The reason is that the surgeons and doctors don't see delirium as one of their top ten things to worry about. It takes a backseat to other critical issues, and that makes sense. So it was up to me to ask about delirium, or research it myself, and I didn't know enough to even ask. I waited too long to advocate for Rick about it.

The cause of his delirium isn't really known, but the best guess was disrupted sleep cycles—he literally didn't sleep for weeks— along with medications, constant complications from surgery and respiratory problems, perhaps withdrawal from his prescribed sleep medications, or maybe even withdrawal from drinking alcohol.

Honestly, his delirium reminded me of reading about POWs who had been physically and mentally tortured by sleep deprivation and constant noise. Rick was insane. I was told he wouldn't remember anything and that he'd get over it. He had vivid hallucinations. He was paranoid, fearful, isolated and antagonized, and the delirium compounded his physical suffering.

It started a few days after his esophagectomy while still in the ICU. Rick asked the nurse in the room with us, "Have you changed the lighting in here?" He thought the walls had turned a bright color.

A few days later he was moved out of the ICU to a step-down unit. When Kelly and I arrived in his new hospital room and met his bedside nurse, Rick was not yet able to swallow. He was given a cup of water with a small sponge to wet his mouth.

As we were sitting around his bed, he seemed normal. I didn't think much about it when he said, "Take a look at my bed. Do you see the bugs?" I just laughed and assured him there were no bugs. But then he wondered about the bugs on the rim of his water cup. That's when I called the nurse, who chuckled somewhat dismissively and explained that he was hallucinating.

"Quite common," she told us. "Don't be alarmed. It will go away."

It didn't go away. And it was alarming him, we realized. Kelly and I talked with him and kept reassuring him that there were no bugs, anywhere.

A day or so later, Rick was taken back to the ICU for the second time, and that evening he took a severe downturn, with escalating delirium that continued for several weeks. He was frightened, seeing rats on the floor under the privacy curtain separating his room from the hallway. He saw a shadow of a man lurking in the corner of the ICU room behind me. I remembered that years earlier Rick had talked with me about his training as a U.S. Navy pilot and how oxygen deprivation causes confusion.

My only instinct was to say to Rick that evening in his darkened room, "You're hallucinating because of the stress on your body and maybe the drugs they're giving you. Remember your pilot training and the confusion that comes with oxygen deprivation, so you might be confused. Trust *me*. Tell me what you see, and I'll let you know if it's real. Rick, I'm right here with you. Don't worry." I explained away the lurking man by identifying and touching a wall-mounted canister, and the scurrying rats under his privacy curtain as the shoes of the passers-by in the hallway.

He was sitting up in a chair in the ICU room, having a hard time breathing, when he confided that he thought he was going to die that night.

"You have the best medical team in America," I reminded him. "We're at Duke Medical Center. Dr. D'Amico and his team and nurses are brilliant. Look out there." I pointed to the large glass sliding door of his room, through which we could partially see the well-lit outside hallway where doctors and nurses were standing. "You have an entire team working to make sure you get better. You're going to get through this. Don't be afraid. We're going to get through this."

A week later he was back in another step-down unit and seemed to have a chance to get better. During Rick's second stay in the unit, he had a bedside nurse named Colby, a Clemson Tiger we all loved, since Kelly was a Clemson graduate. She took good care of Rick. She informed me one night that he'd been given a sleep medication that caused him to awaken thinking he was in danger. He'd tried to pull out the lines and tubes from his body and escape from the threat, calling out to those around him to follow him into the woods. Colby and others calmed him down by asking him questions like, "How old are you?"

"Nineteen years old," he responded.

Late the following night, when Rick couldn't sleep again, Colby took him by wheelchair to another floor that had a giant aquarium. It delighted him. She took photos of him on his iPhone so she could show us how much pleasure that aquarium gave him—such a compassionate gesture on her part to give Rick, and us, a moment or two of relief. Go, Tigers!

A few days later he aspirated digestive fluid into his lungs and quickly began experiencing respiratory failure. It was back to the ICU for the third time.

Weeks went by. He had critical complications, going on and off the ventilator for about three weeks, enduring one stressful event after another to his mind and body. No real rest, no sleep, week after week.

Rick was finally off the ventilator, but his delirium persisted. He'd now had delirium for about eight weeks. He thought he was in a hotel. He thought he had been in a helicopter crash and was in a hospital in Cleveland. He kept asking me who that woman was standing beside me, when nobody else was in the room. He described her pink dress. He confided to me that the physicians were all conspiring against him with tests and treatments that weren't necessary. He was paranoid. Fearful. I just kept talking to him, telling him that the doctors and nurses were on our side and he was getting better.

And much worse were his middle-of-the-night phone calls to me. I still have some of the messages. In a voice I'd never heard in our 34 years together, Rick cried, "Kim Norris, where are you?!" He was in the third-floor basement and couldn't get out, he said, and there were people making noise so they couldn't hear him call out. He sounded so desperate.

I would call the night nurse and ask them to look in on him, and to turn off the TV in case it was contributing to his lack of sleep and hallucinations. I didn't know what to do. All I knew was that my brave husband was now fearful, hallucinating, isolated and calling out for me in the predawn hours to help him.

Early on, Rick had been given medication that I did not see as helpful. Here's what I finally did:

Around June 10, 2018, Rick was placed in a step-down unit for the third time. He'd been suffering delirium for almost two months. After getting the second consecutive incoherent call from my frightened husband in the predawn hours, I called his nurse and asked that the surgery fellow on duty from Dr. D'Amico's team call me. It was the middle of the night, adding to my unpopular "reputation."

The fellow did call, but he was not that happy to speak with me, to say the least. It was the middle of the night, so he was probably exhausted like the rest of us and had way too much to do. Delirium was not at the top of his list of concerns. But I told him about Rick's desperate phone calls anyway. Here's basically how my end of the conversation went:

"My husband has been delirious for about eight weeks now. I'm not a medical professional, but my common sense tells me *his medication is not working*! What is your plan to review his meds? What can be done and when?"

A psychiatric consult happened on June 14. The three psych evaluators saw Rick, then stood out in the hall to talk with me.

They asked questions and listened intently as I related how long he'd been like this and described his delirium as best I could.

Weeks earlier, the ICU nurses counseled me that sunlight and being back in touch with his normal life would help him get over the delirium. The nurses, sometimes two or three at a time, labored to get Rick into a wheelchair, or would literally wheel his bed into the hallway for sunlight or just a change of scenery, hoping to alleviate the delirium.

Now that he was out of the ICU, I lobbied the psychiatrists for permission to wheelchair Rick out of his step-down hospital room to a window, or even outside in the courtyard for air and sun, for a few minutes each day.

What they said was music to my ears. "You're right. His medication isn't working, and we've recommended a new one to help him out of the delirium. It will take a couple of days. And yes, getting him out in the sun and air will help. We'll work with the nurses to have field trips and do them safely."

Within a few days, Kelly and I could see Rick was getting better—no more calls for help at night, no more men lurking in the shadows. It was a bit of a slow climb back; but by June 25, he was "speaking in a reality-based way," the medical record noted. By July 2 he was back to reality.

I must admit, there were times we couldn't help but laugh while he was coming out of the worst of his delirium. He would react to whatever was on the TV in his room. His personality was surfacing to our enjoyment, like insisting we all go on vacation to the Bahamas (in response to TV ads), making sure to invite anyone he came into contact with. Kelly was instructed to make hotel and air reservations for all of us.

Our dear friend Jim Cawley flew in from New Jersey to spend the afternoon with him. I'll never forget how happy Rick was to see his friend, calling out in an excited voice as he saw him round the corner, "*Jiiiimmmmm!*" and then playing music from his iPhone in the room as if we were partying in the back yard.

On another day his Michigan State University fraternity brother Jim Jackson flew in and brought photos of their lifelong friendship, bringing back good memories for Rick. Close friend Brad White called many times from Dallas and had long, uplifting conversation with him. Contact with them was such a great help in bringing my husband back.

While watching Fox News cover a congressional hearing and the excoriation of a witness, Rick became a congressman, ringing the nurse assistance button.

"This is Congressman Norris. Could you come in, please?"

Without missing a beat, the receptionist replied, "Yes, Mr. Norris, someone will be right there."

I would say, "Rick, you're not a congressman."

He'd smile at my ignorance and reply, "Yes, I am."

We all had a good laugh.

While watching a major golf tournament on TV, he thought he was an actual participant. As the young doctors would come in and out of the room, he'd invite them to join him for the next round. The doctors were very nice, saying they'd love to but couldn't because they had to "go back to work" and weren't very good golfers anyway.

Seeing him come out of the depths with some lighthearted conversations and comments was such a relief. We were able to laugh, and we knew things were going to get better. He even sent me a dozen roses and a love note through our daughter while he was coming out of his delirium. That's my Rick, the love of my life.

LESSONS LEARNED

- None of the physicians I interviewed saw ICU delirium as one of their top ten concerns, which explains why nobody mentioned it to me up front. It's not seen as particularly life-threatening from the doctor's perspective. But the bedside nurses see it every day and know how troubling it is for the families to witness.

- Being able to describe what I'd seen over the past several weeks helped me advocate for Rick, and the psychiatry professionals listened instead of minimizing my observations.

- It would have been more productive to speak with the bedside nurses on a regular basis about my concern over Rick's delirium. With their help, I would have been able to advocate more regularly for a medication plan.

- Once back home, Rick very vaguely remembered his frightening delirium episodes. But from what I've read, delirium can lead to dementia-like issues once the patient is out of the hospital. It's fair to say Rick was not the same person when he finally came home, but he was well enough to enjoy a few months of peace.

- When Rick was about to be discharged to an inpatient rehab hospital, I asked the Duke psychiatry clinician what I should know about his Risperdal medication. She told me that the physicians in the rehab hospital would likely keep him on the medication for too long, and it wasn't necessary. She gave me a 10-day time frame. If the physician had not started to take him off by then, I should speak up about it. I later found out that it was very good advice.

TIPS FROM THE WHITE COATS TO HELP WITH DELIRIUM

- Preserve the sleep cycle as much as possible. During the day, try to stay awake. At night, turn off the TV, darken the room, ask for quiet and try to sleep.

- Try to have a window in the hospital room or go on a field trip to be near a window during the day.

- When a patient is unpredictable and needs someone constantly around, a trained "sitter" can be assigned through the nursing team. But it helps a patient sleep if a familiar person is in the room at night. If the family advocates are available, it's comforting to the patient for an advocate to stay with them overnight, instead of a hospital sitter.

- Family members and visitors can do wonders to help keep the patient grounded in reality. While they try to keep the patient awake during the day, music, conversation, card-playing, other games or something as simple as their touch make a difference.

- Allow for a short nap during the day if the patient is very tired, but only for an hour or so. I would encourage Rick to take an hour's nap by bringing the large reclining chair alongside his bed and touching his arm or hand, or placing my feet next to him, and saying, "Let's take a nap." Kind of like we'd done throughout our thirty-four years together.

- Bring in white noise or calming sounds to encourage sleep at night. Find the "white noise" channel on the hospital TV. It's there!

Vanderbilt University has been studying ICU delirium for nearly twenty years and is a part of the Critical Illness, Brain Dysfunction and Survivorship (CIBS) Center. Dr. Wes Ely, a pulmonologist and professor of medicine and critical care at Vanderbilt University Medical Center in Nashville, Tennessee, considers ICU delirium a "massive public health problem."

Again, I'm certainly no expert on delirium, so if you seek further information, a good start would be a search for the article titled "Delirium in the intensive care unit," which was published May 14, 2008, in the journal *Critical Care*. Other helpful works include the STAT News article "Hospitals struggle to address terrifying and long-lasting ICU delirium," published on October 14, 2016, and Vanderbilt University's "New center formed to treat, study ICU delirium, dementia," published Oct. 4, 2018.

CHAPTER SEVEN

Friends, Faith and Gifts

FRIENDS

I was beyond fortunate to be on the receiving end of uplifting well wishes and support from friends and family, even strangers, during our health crisis. It sounds almost a trite thing to say, but it's heartfelt, I assure you. I include this chapter simply to share lessons I've learned about the power of giving and compassion. People who gave of their time, kindness, love and energy—in ways that may have seemed small to them—buoyed and bolstered us during the turmoil. Their acts were profound reminders of the critical importance that generosity of spirit plays in healing and comforting others.

Many, many times, our friends saved us. Whether facing troubles of their own such as grave medical circumstances or enjoying well-earned, happy lives, our extended family set aside time to think of and care for us. I want to be that kind of human being.

Their actions illustrate how compassion accumulates to create a wave of good. For us as receivers of their attention and care, their collective compassion created a river of gratitude that flowed back to each of them—though perhaps not nearly as well expressed as they deserve.

To this day, I'm inspired by our South Carolina neighbors who knew us for only a year, in some cases just a few months, before this all started, and made us feel loved—and never alone.

If not for neighborhood friends Michael Franck and Will Miller, I'm not sure what we would have done. They exemplify the level of grace and kindness to which we should all aspire. We'd known one another for a short time, yet they were incredibly supportive throughout Rick's yearlong ordeal and were helpful in so many ways it's difficult to describe properly. Michael and Will took care of our leased home for three months, and in a hundred different ways assured us that we were in their minds and hearts. During Rick's final weeks of life, they helped us move into a new residence, stocking the kitchen with food and arranging furniture in the living space so that we'd have a place to rest after returning from Rick's second hospitalization at Duke. And, so much more …

Most profound was the spiritual assistance given by Michael and Will. After Rick's passing, I was dazed with grief. They literally took me by the hand and led me to join their church, which brought about our important connection with The Reverend Michael S. White, Rector of Christ Church in Savannah.

Michael White delivered a wonderful memorial service for Rick in a small chapel along the May River. He also helped me make sense of things by telling me about "thin places," a Celtic Christian term for "those rare locales where the distance between Heaven and Earth collapses"—in other words, where the veil between this world and the next is thin, where one may experience things that seem outside of normal, otherworldly.

Our Bluffton neighbors were like warrior angels. Stan and Erin Pennington, whom we knew for only a few months before all this happened, did the laborious heavy-lifting of unpacking several rooms of our moving boxes that were practically stacked to the ceiling. They set up our master bedroom in the newly purchased house. Erin put our bed together, while Olivia, their beautiful 9-year-old daughter, made sure our clothes and shoes were properly unpacked. Little brother Max helped by saying bedtime prayers for Rick. Stan, with a wink, set the TV remote to Rick's favorite Fox News channel. The Pennington family: a force of nature.

There were continuous sweet gifts and flowers from my friend Carol. During our tough times at Duke, the kind, supportive messages she sent were so touching that I find it difficult to read them to this day.

Our New Jersey friend, Philip Rushton, happened to be in Savannah for a business meeting and came to check on us during our harried move to our Remington Road home. Rick was settled in a hotel room just minutes away while I moved into our new house, running back and forth to check on him throughout the day. Philip was in my car when, by speakerphone, Scott Balderson, Dr. D'Amico's P.A., with whom I'd been in close contact, implored me to drop everything and get Rick to the ER at Duke, five hours away. I was completely overwhelmed.

Philip had me pull the car to the side of Old Moreland Road and told me to leave for Duke *"right now."* He would handle the move from here and calmly took charge. Philip checked in by phone during our five-hour drive that afternoon. He calmed me down with his charming British banter and spoke to Rick as if we were on a Sunday afternoon tour of the countryside instead of a dreadful journey. Thank you, Philip.

Rick's lifelong friends saved us. Throughout his hospitalization, they appeared at Rick's hospital bedside. Our dear friend from New Jersey, Hillary Smith, traveled to Rick's ICU bedside multiple times, breaking through to her bedridden and delirious friend for minutes at a time by playing cards with him, and encouraging him while he worked hard to form the words "get my shoes," because "we're going home."

Jim Jackson, Rick's lifelong friend and fraternity brother from Michigan State University flew in from Michigan; Jim Cawley from New Jersey flew in to spend the day; Tom and Joy Jackson, lifelong friends from Florida, came several times; and Brad White, another close friend, called in from Texas with one encouraging conversation after another.

Our daughter's friends in Raleigh were an amazing group of Millennials. They showed up to Kelly and Stephen's apartment with dinners, and Maggie especially, took time to cheerfully visit with me over dinner. Kelly's church community, who did not know my husband or me at all, provided for us and prayed for us. If any of you have ever worried about American's future, don't. The Millennials are an amazing generation. Knowing the future of this world is in their capable, kind and loving hands should give us all hope.

Our daughters Carolyn and Kelly, and our son-in-law Stephen, were incredible. As Rick's hospital stay lasted one, two, three months, my stress and lack of sleep were sometimes a bit much. Imagine having your mother-in-law unexpectedly live with you and stress out in your apartment for three months and being cheerful about it: That's what a good guy Stephen is. Our family was the safe harbor.

Rick and I felt those waves of love and energy sent from near and far, creating hope that washed over us in the worst of times, always letting us know we were not alone, and that we were loved. We were undeservedly fortunate to have this support and are grateful beyond words for the blessing of their friendship.

FAITH

Rick's three-month stay at Duke University Hospital felt like a battle.

We started out knowing nothing about how brutal his recovery could be, or how to navigate the hospital system. Kelly and I learned as we went along.

After about a month of witnessing Rick's suffering, it all became too much. We knew he was enduring this suffering to stay with us.

One evening I'd returned home from the hospital and, as had become my routine, tried to rest before my 10 p.m. call to the night nurse. But this night, brokenhearted and overcome with sorrow, for the first time since I was a little girl, in the privacy of my bedroom, I got on my knees at the bedside like my mother taught me.

I prayed to God in total submission, with all my heart and laid everything at His feet. My prayer is between myself and the Almighty, but part of it was this:

> "Sorrow is overtaking me. I was wrong to think I could take on this battle without You. I'm grateful for all the blessings You've given, please forgive my disregard of Your love and Your word. I was so wrong. I pray for forgiveness, for strength to care for Rick. Help him recover. Please... have mercy on Rick and help me care for him."

We all may experience such an intimate moment, when only one's faith can conquer an overwhelming sense of dread. After my prayer, I was better able to see God's presence all around us, grace in the ordinary, the quiet, the extra effort, mercy in music and in the joyful expression of kindness. Providing what is needed with perfect timing, given through strangers and friends, and I'm convinced... angels.

So, I want to share a few examples with you, because it may give you hope as it did for me.

GIFTS ALONG THE WAY

Read Poem

In rare moments of peace that Rick had in the ICU, when he wasn't on a ventilator and could speak, he'd tell me how much he loved our South Carolina home.

"I want to go home ... I want to walk down to the dock ... Let's go home now ... When we get back home, we're going to retire and enjoy life more ..."

I'd promise him we would; but truthfully, sorrowfully, I doubted that he'd ever go home. In the dark night, things seemed so bleak. Only prayer gave me hope.

There were a few times when Rick was able to cheerfully greet me as I walked into his ICU room. During our thirty-four years together, Rick teased that he'd spent half his life waiting for me. One morning in the ICU he was sitting up slightly in his bed when I arrived.

"Well, hello, Kim Norris. You made it!" (Translation: I was late, and he'd been waiting.)

I put my arms around him and whispered, "Wild horses couldn't drag me away from you, my sweetheart."

He murmured back, "Young and beautiful ..." to his haggard six-ty-six-year-old wife. "... Young and beautiful ... "

Rick was now about four weeks in the ICU. It was mid May, 2018, and he'd been on the ventilator for about a week at this point. The medication to keep Rick somewhat awake yet sedated while on the respirator had to be consistently balanced. He would wake up a bit and I would catch his eye.

The nurses talked with me each day about the medication and said that Rick could hear us. They would explain how important it was, when he was not being closely watched, to keep his wrists loosely bound with soft restraints just enough so he could not reach the ventilator breathing tube. If Rick were alone and the meds were not balanced, he may try to pull the ventilator tubes out.

Sometimes he'd look at me with tears welling up. I knew he was suffering and fearful, and I could only reassure him that I was with him, I loved him, and he was going to get better.

One day while intubated on the ventilator, Kelly and I were at his bedside. Rick was calm and surfaced a little, kind of awake, and wanted to communicate with us. He'd raise his right hand to panto-mime "writing." Kelly asked if he wanted to write on a whiteboard, and he nodded yes. We handed him a small whiteboard and marker. He tried his best to write, but it was just scribbling. He kept trying until he wrote these words: "Call police."

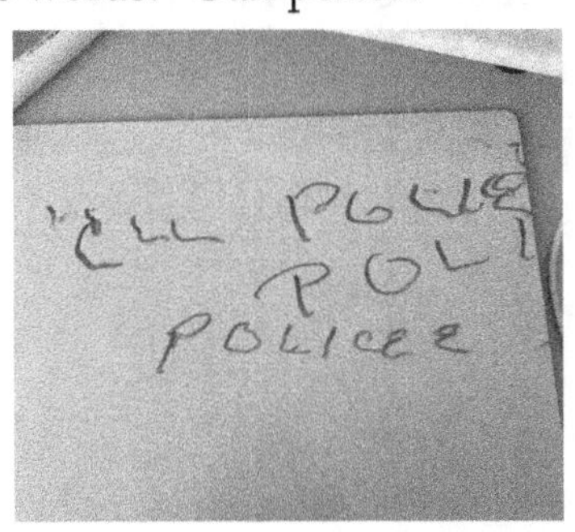

It was like Rick to want to protect us. Kelly and I assured him that everything was okay, we were okay, and so was he. There was no need to call the police right now, but we would do as he told us if necessary. *Trust us.*

That evening we left just after the night nurse started her shift report. Rick seemed to be sleeping. I couldn't speak with the new nurse, so I decided I'd call later and went back to Raleigh.

At about 11 p.m. his very pleasant nurse was free to speak, and I could feel her reassuring presence through the phone. She said she'd been "chatting" with Rick, and he had made her laugh. Of course, he was still intubated and could not speak, but I knew what she meant—he'd been communicating with her.

He'd motioned with his hand, she told me, indicating that he wanted to write. She watched him write "read poem" on the small white board. How unlike him to want to read poetry, since spy novels were more his thing. The nurse had apologized to "Mr. Norris" for having no poems to read, but he kept tapping the words "read poem" on the board and moving his head as if to say, "Yes... read poem." She was sweet enough to comment on how charming and engaging Rick was, even though he was intubated. Yes, I knew exactly what she meant.

The next day a big care package was delivered to the Raleigh apartment from our South Carolina friends. I opened it that evening when I returned from Duke and found it was filled with cards, delightful gifts and goodies ... and a small book of poems.

The book is titled "The Four Seasons - Poems." The inside cover read:

"Everyman,
I will go with thee

and be thy guide,
in thy most need
to go by thy side."

A slender yellow ribbon marked page 101, featuring the poem "Summer Wind," by William Cullen Bryant:

"It is a sultry day; the sun has drunk
The dew that lay upon the morning grass.
There is no rustling in the lofty elm
That canopies my dwelling and its shade
Scarce cools me..."

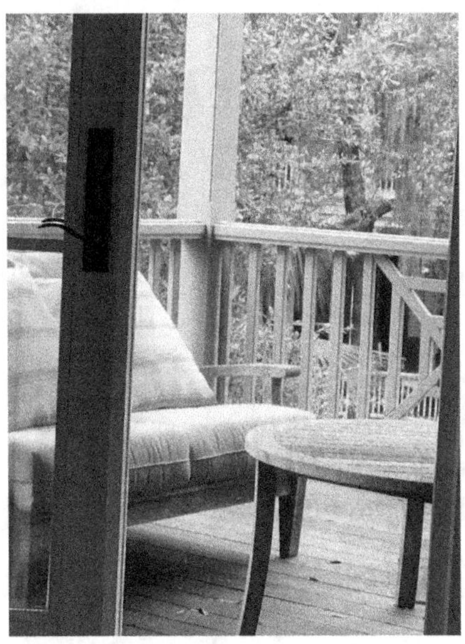

The words struck me—"the lofty elm that canopies my dwelling." I immediately saw our second-floor bedroom porch that was very much like a tree house, it was so canopied by trees. A bedroom that we longed for ... to rest there together again.

Many a night Rick and I had been in bed with the doors wide open to the fresh air, whispering to each other. "It's like being in a big tree house... so restful... the birds... " There was sometimes a faint, lovely fragrance of the May River only a short block away. It was the most wonderful bedroom.

So I took this to be the poem Rick wanted us to read, a message that he would be home in the summer. I believe it was a message of love and mercy from God, reminding me that there is a plan.

My friend Erin, who had selected the items in the care package, told me the book just happened to be something she thought was pleasant ... and she herself had not placed the ribbon marker.

Rick did indeed finally come home that summer, on July 20, and did find a few months of peace on the second-floor porch canopied by trees. On September 26, we were able to make his victory walk to the neighborhood dock on the May River that Rick had so desperately yearned for while in the ICU, the serene May River, with its magical dolphins and beautiful water fowl, and friends nearby ...

Invisible

As Rick was nearing his eighth week in the ICU, his respiratory issues were getting better. He no longer needed a ventilator, but he was very weak and continued to be delirious. Supported by the nurses, Rick was finally getting out of the ICU on field trips to the outside.

One Friday, in the late afternoon, Rick's nurse Bethlehem sat him up in a wheelchair with the help of a nurse assistant Anthony, a smart, strapping young man with shoulder length dreadlocks. Rick always remembered Anthony whenever he came by. Although Anthony said it was his dreads that made him memorable, we all knew it was so much more. Anthony always made time to talk to Rick like a man. Rick had been so surrounded by women ... which, rest assured, he loved ... but talking with Anthony became a treat for him. Rick truly enjoyed and needed Anthony's energy and conversation.

With Rick in a wheelchair, Anthony, Bethlehem and I set out on a field trip to the lovely courtyard beside Duke's Medical Pavilion. Very few people were around as we sat down at an outdoor table. But there was a small gathering of maybe a half dozen students seated at a nearby table, listening to a speaker.

Rick thought he was in a hospital in Cleveland and had been in a helicopter crash. He even remembered the walls crashing down on him. He was still confused when I told him he was at Duke, but it didn't really matter because he was just so happy to be outside, and he spontaneously called out to the gathering of young nurses, "Hi! Come join us!" They ignored him, and he looked a little dejected.

Anthony moved to a chair closer to Rick and began chatting with him. Rick had been isolated for about two months, and we all knew he was hungry to socialize, hungry for human contact.

Rick was still weak, so the outing had to be limited, and Bethlehem decided it was time for him to go back to the ICU. She and I walked behind Anthony, who was pushing Rick's wheelchair as we headed back inside to the elevator.

It was late in the day, and the hallway was almost empty, with just an occasional person passing by as we walked along.

Then Rick spotted a man coming up the hallway and called out, "Hi! How are you?" as the man passed by ignoring Rick's shout out. Then, in his confused state, Rick said aloud to himself, "I think I'm invisible."

Anthony quickly corrected him. "No, man, you're not invisible. We're gonna try again."

A couple came walking toward us. Their two young children, who looked to be maybe 6 and 8, were taking a leisurely stroll behind them. The man and the woman ignored Rick's "Hi!" as they passed him. He tried again when the children came by, saying hi and waving to them. The younger child, a precious little girl, stopped. Her face lit up in the most radiant smile, and she joyously, enthusiastically, waved back to Rick with the most playful, "Hi! Hi! Hi!"

To which Anthony remarked, "See, Rick, you thought you were invisible. You are not invisible, man."

Such an extraordinary gift of kindness from Anthony and the little girl to a man who'd been so isolated by illness and delirium, so starved for human touch, that for a moment he really did think he was invisible. It took a child and one good man to lift him up again.

Desperado

Within the first few days of Rick's surgery on April 16, 2018, he was recovering in his ICU room when a young man, a guitarist, walked in and greeted us. Duke Hospital has a program where musicians play throughout the hospital for the enjoyment of the patients and families, a lovely, healing gesture by this wonderful medical center.

The guitarist asked if Rick had a request. Being an Eagles fan, Rick asked for his favorite song, "Desperado." The guitarist seemed a bit caught off guard, apologizing that he didn't really know the lyrics and explaining that he never gets that song as a request, so he was a bit rusty. The young man tried but didn't know the song. It was a nice try, we thanked him, and he moved along to the next patient.

Now fast-forward several weeks to early June. Rick no longer needed the ventilator as of June 1 but was still in the ICU, in his sixth week. We were all hoping to help break his delirium with field trips, but it was difficult.

One day, a young man poked his head in Rick's ICU room, asking for Mr. Norris. Rick was sitting in a wheelchair next to me as I invited the young man to come in, and only then did I recognize the guitarist we'd met in April.

"Back in April I didn't do such a good job remembering the lyrics to 'Desperado,'" he reminded us. "Since then it seems I've had requests for 'Desperado' two or three times a week throughout the hospital, so I've learned the lyrics and was hoping to find Mr. Norris and sing it for him." I couldn't believe it!

Rick was sitting next to me in a wheelchair, struggling with confusion and delirium, not communicating very well.

The guitarist began to play, and sing so sweetly:

"Desperado,
Why don't you come to your senses
You've been out ridin' fences
For so long now.
Oh, you're a hard one,
But I know that you've got your reasons.
These things that are pleasin' you
Can hurt you somehow."

When the guitarist launched into the chorus, Rick joined in, with a strong and joyful voice! It was as if he was back to reality and, for a few minutes, enjoying himself.

"Don't you draw the queen of diamonds, boy,
She'll beat you if she's able.

You know the queen of hearts is always your best bet ..."

It's well known that music can be miraculous in its ability to connect human beings and bring up life memories, especially for those who are struggling medically. What a gift from this kind young musician who returned to find Rick and sing his favorite song, just when we needed him. He could easily have forgotten about Rick during those several weeks, but he remembered, and delivered a magnificent gift.

$1.89 ... Hero

It was now later in June. Rick was in a step-down unit, still struggling with delirium and confusion. We continued going on field trips, hoping to help him come back to reality.

One day, with Rick in a wheelchair, we rode the elevator down to the main lobby of Duke Hospital. It was busy, with lots of activity everywhere—a piano playing, lots of people in the waiting area, other people coming and going at the bank of filled elevators, people on their way to the cafeteria, more people moving around in the sunny, tree-shaded courtyard visible through the wall of windows.

We moved through the hustle and bustle between the elevators and the waiting area and passed a small gift shop. The doors were open, and a rack hung on one of them, displaying nail clippers and other small grooming items. As we passed by, Rick, in his wheelchair, with his IV and nurse assistant, announced, "I need the fingernail clippers. Can't find my clippers in the room." I assured him that when we returned to his room, I'd come back to get them, but I didn't have my purse with me. He persisted, not in a loud, dramatic way, just conversationally explaining how important the clippers were.

"Just tell the gift shop to put it on our room tab," he instructed, because he thought we were in a hotel.

The clippers cost something like $1.89. I reluctantly took them from the rack, left Rick with the nurse, stepped a few paces into the gift shop through a group gathered around the array of snacks, and approached the lovely volunteer at the cash register. "My husband needs these clippers, and I didn't bring my pocketbook with me for his walk. May I please give them to him and come back in a few minutes with the money?"

Before she could respond, I felt a hand on my shoulder. It was a man, a total stranger, who quietly said, "Please let me pay for the clippers. It would be my pleasure. In fact, I insist." He opened his well-worn wallet that had just a few bills in it and paid for Rick's nail clippers. It was such a touching act of kindness, and I accepted his gift with humble gratitude. His kindness is something I'll always remember.

CHAPTER EIGHT

Advocating for Discharge and Inpatient Rehabilitation

IMPORTANT: ADVOCATING TO THE DISCHARGE PLANNER

This chapter is based on conversations with Sandra Bond, who at the time of this interview, was the executive director of a well-known hospice organization, and, Renee Bannon, who is the business development director at Encompass Health Rehabilitation Hospital of Bluffton.

From the moment any patient is admitted into a hospital, there is a person dedicated to planning for the discharge, and this preparation begins immediately. Until our Duke Hospital experience, I had no clue about how important the discharge plan could be to Rick's recovery. And more importantly, I had no idea how critical it was to advocate for the *right* discharge plan.

Of course, it makes sense. The hospital needs to keep patients moving from the emergency room, the operating rooms, progressive care units and acute care units—everything has to filter through the hospital to control bottlenecks and keep the patients flowing. Many hospitals will have a long wait for an ICU room when admitted through the ER. This happened to us at Savannah Memorial Hospital. Discharge planning keeps things moving.

Discharge planners have different titles. For us, the case manager planned Rick's discharge. Her job was to release Rick from the hospital to the appropriate next stage of care or service—whether home care, a skilled nursing home, an inpatient rehabilitation hospital or hospice. I experienced that she needed to be engaged and encouraged to help find the right next step for Rick.

This is very important: The discharge planner, or case manager, will have a long list of patients to release each day, let's say 25 patients. They will do the easiest things possible that fit the patients' needs.

Release to home care is the easiest. Less paperwork and less explanation. What takes more time and effort is finding the best inpatient rehabilitation hospital, or talking about hospice options, or looking for a good skilled nursing facility.

Discharge planners are often relieved when there is no advocate or family member participating in the discharge plan—nobody there to add complications to an already overwhelming job. To get the best next stage of care after being released from the hospital, the advocate has to understand *all the available options* so that they can have informed discussions with the case manager early in the hospital stay. And for us that meant showing up to visit proposed facilities before agreeing to have our loved one placed.

INPATIENT REHABILITATION HOSPITAL

As mentioned earlier, physical therapy was critical to Rick's recovery while he was hospitalized. Just about everyone who's had a critical illness and a long hospital stay will need physical, occupational or speech therapy when they are discharged. The question is, where will this care take place: a skilled nursing facility (referred to as SNF), an inpatient rehabilitation hospital (often referred to as IRF, for inpatient rehabilitation facility), or home?

It was critical that Rick have the highest level of rehabilitative care possible in order to recover after all he had endured. He was very weak from being so ill and bedridden for almost three months and battling delirium for almost as long. The better the rehabilitation, the better the recovery, and the better the quality of life for Rick when he returned home.

My experience may be different than yours, but I learned that planning rehabilitation care is best done a week or so before discharge actually takes place. It's difficult to understand discharge planning in advance, but the advocate must make it an issue well before discharge. The more you understand the options, the better the chances that your loved one will be placed in the right facility for rehabilitation.

I found that the burden to locate superior care and push for it was up to me, as Rick's advocate. Hospital physicians and case managers will not recommend a facility, because showing "favoritism" is not allowed.

The status quo unfortunately seems to be discharge to home or placement in a skilled nursing facility, unless someone advocates for the highest possible level of care. Often the inpatient rehabilitation hospitals and skilled nursing facilities are lumped together as if they are the same. They are *not* the same. Inpatient rehabilitation hospitals are far superior to skilled nursing facilities in terms of rehabilitation.

Of course, there are perfectly good skilled nursing facilities that benefit particular patients. However, the facilities we toured did not hold up to an inpatient rehabilitation hospital in terms of providing a well-rounded program to set the patient up to return home. It was obvious to me that superior rehabilitation was in the inpatient rehabilitation hospital setting. This was also affirmed for me in a scientific statement comparing the two types of facilities, issued by the American Heart Association/American Stroke Association in 2018.

Inpatient Rehabilitation Hospital vs. Skilled Nursing Facility

1. Physician participation in patient therapy and medical care.

    A PM&R physician, or physiatrist, is available full time in the inpatient rehabilitation hospital. PM&R stands for "physical medicine and rehabilitation." It's a medical specialty. A physiatrist is a medical doctor who specializes in physical medicine, rehabilitation and pain medicine. This kind of doctor will prescribe a therapy program and monitor and manage the patient's medical needs as well. The total patient is the focus. A skilled nursing facility has no such doctor on site full time.

    Per today's Medicare guidelines, for example, at a minimum, the physiatrist in an inpatient rehabilitation hospital is required to round three times a week on each patient, whereas a physician in a skilled nursing facility is required to see patients only once a month. This is a big difference in care.

2. Patients required to achieve therapy goals.

In an inpatient rehabilitation hospital, patients must have three hours per day of therapy: physical, occupational or speech therapy combined. Or, if they need to work up to the therapy goals, they can do fifteen hours of combined therapy over seven days. But patient participation is required, whereas in a skilled nursing facility, therapy offered is usually one hour per day, or sometimes shorter.

This patient participation requirement means that patients being discharged, like my husband, must be well enough to tolerate the therapy goals. This can be tricky. Rick was declined admittance to the first inpatient rehabilitation hospital we wanted in Raleigh.

Here is where you must work with the medical team prior to discharge to be sure your loved one is ready for the higher level of rehabilitative care. I'll share my experience in the next section.

Our Discharge Experience

It was the last week of June 2018. My husband was to be discharged within the week. Yet, he was frail. He could only stand and walk for a few minutes and needed help with the activities of daily living. Being an inpatient at Duke Hospital was soon to be no longer called for from a medical standpoint; but having been alongside him every day of those eleven inpatient weeks, I knew he had a long way to go before I could take care of him at home.

The case manager gave me several printed pages—which she got off the internet—of about thirty rehabilitation hospitals and nursing homes in the Raleigh-Durham area. She declined to recommend any of them, because she said it was illegal for her to do so. I would have to choose one for myself.

Her inability to recommend a facility for Rick's care was not helpful. Here is where the patient and advocates should be offered an opportunity to meet with representatives from rehabilitation hospitals or hospice providers while still hospitalized. That would help the advocate and patient be well informed about all options and work with the medical team for a successful recovery.

My daughter Kelly and I narrowed down the list to about ten facilities in the Raleigh-Durham area and set out one day to appear, unannounced, at each one to see how things looked. There is no substitute for showing up in person for the sights and the smells of these facilities. What an eye-opener. Many places will break your heart.

I've since learned that the best time to appear unannounced at inpatient rehabilitation hospitals, memory care facilities, skilled nursing facilities, or assisted living facilities is on weekends, holidays and at night: not during daytime business hours.

We did find one fantastic inpatient rehab hospital in Raleigh that we thought could be a perfect fit. It would have been a three-week stay with focus on physical, occupational and speech therapy, and general recovery. As noted, one morning I appeared unannounced, was taken on a tour by a very capable employee and saw the workout areas, the bedrooms, the entire facility. I listened as a patient in a wheelchair, alongside me in the elevator, received kind words of encouragement from an attentive young physical therapist. I cried when I walked out of the facility that day, thinking Rick would be given a real opportunity there to get better and come home.

I returned to Duke Hospital to speak with the case manager and surgery fellow in charge. The three of us stood in the hallway outside my husband's hospital room in the step-down unit.

The conversation was basically this: Rick did not meet the requirements of that Raleigh rehabilitation hospital because of his lingering delirium and PT assessments, and he would have to be placed in one of the local skilled nursing facilities.

I responded with something like, "I have personally toured those facilities, and I will not allow my husband to be warehoused. If he's not ready to be released, then to you (looking at the case manager) and to your team (looking at the Fellow) I have to ask: Have you done your very best? His delirium is getting better, and he needs just a little more time. What can be done? We *all* need to do our very best!"

To be fair, there are insurance concerns to be taken into consideration as well as patient flow. The inpatient rehabilitation hospitals select new patients based on PT assessments and whether or not the patient can achieve certain PT levels of rehabilitation. It's not as easy as it looks for someone like Rick, who was on the cusp of getting better. But I found that if more is asked of the medical professionals around you, they will help you. As an advocate, the question I always ended up asking myself was, *"Have we done our very best?"*

Because of a combination of issues, Rick was given a few more days to respond to PT assessments. His delirium kept getting a bit better, and the case manager dug into where we might find another option for him.

This ultimately led us to Encompass Health Rehabilitation Hospital of Bluffton, South Carolina, a brand-new inpatient hospital just twenty minutes from our home. Although I had not visited the facility, I could tell from their website and conversations with the case manager that it was a lot like the Raleigh hospital. It was absolutely the best opportunity for Rick, and he was accepted into their hospital thanks to the case manager working with the PT and medical team.

He ended up staying for the full 21-day program and was much stronger when he came home. We were both well trained on things like going up and down stairs, walking outside in the neighborhood, eating, dressing and bathing. Before releasing Rick, the therapy team did a dry run for us, going on a field trip to our home one morning to see for themselves the layout of our house and then training us to overcome the physical obstacles at home, like steep staircases.

The right rehabilitation program enabled Rick to enjoy a much better quality of life when he was finally discharged on July 20, 2018. He was able to use a walker to finally stroll around the neighborhood, a goal that kept him going. For a few precious months he was able to eat and drink some of his favorites, although small amounts; visit with family and neighbors; and just have a few months of peace.

It was well worth advocating for.

Advice from the Professionals,
Renee Bannon and Sandra Bond

- It's important to ask the medical team when you should be planning for discharge. Other questions you should ask:

   "What kind of therapy is going to be prescribed?"

   "How can we plan for my loved one to meet the requirements for an inpatient rehabilitation hospital instead of a skilled nursing facility?"

   "What should I be looking for in terms of therapy offered in an inpatient rehabilitation hospital?"

- Share with the discharge planner your needs and questions, for example:

   "I'd like to talk with a hospice representative now in case it becomes an option for us."

   "When can my husband be discharged? I'll need to be sure care services are lined up."

   "I'd like to discuss the details of the release plan."

- In terms of rehabilitation, status quo seems to be placing patients in a skilled nursing home first. If this happens, seek a second opinion, because an inpatient rehabilitation hospital has the superior outcome for most people. It's worthwhile to advocate for the option that will offer the better quality of life.

Don't hesitate to ask the case manager for the best facility. "I expect you to help find the best possible inpatient rehab hospital for my loved one. What is your plan?"

- It was critical to have invested time in personally visiting inpatient rehabilitation hospitals, rehabilitation facilities and nursing homes before agreeing to let Rick be placed in any of them.

- When you hear "It can't be done," or "You'll have to do X," respectfully ask "Why?" as many times as necessary if enough information isn't provided about the plan.

CHAPTER NINE

Home Health Care

You may have an altogether different journey than ours, but hopefully, there will come a time when your loved one is able to return home. Many times, by necessity, home health care then becomes the next phase of recovery.

In our case, after 11 weeks of hospitalization, Rick was finally discharged from Duke Hospital to Encompass Health Rehabilitation Hospital of Bluffton, South Carolina, for another 3 weeks of in-patient rehabilitation therapy. After the 3-week rehabilitation, to prepare for discharge from Encompass, an in-home team of PT specialists were set up to continue his care. They trained both of us which enabled Rick to continue to get better. With help, he was able to dress, walk up and down steep stairs, go outside for a neighborhood stroll using his walker, visit with friends in the living room, and enjoy tiny portions of his favorite food and water and tea several times a day. This went on for almost three months, and Rick seemed to be gaining strength. His skin returned to a healthy color, and he seemed to be enjoying himself a little. It felt like a victory… a miracle.

We eventually hired an in-home caregiver to watch over Rick during the day. Like everything else, you have to advocate for good caregivers.

Finding the right in-home care of an elderly or ill person is difficult. It takes patience, commitment to training the caregiver once they're in your home, and constant observation until it's safe to leave your vulnerable loved one alone with them. No matter what, don't leave your loved one at home alone with the caregiver unless you've got a real sense of confidence, and even then, return home unexpectedly at times. Keep a watchful eye for signs of neglect. Cameras are a good idea. Unfortunately, the reality is that the vulnerable are easy prey.

In-home care franchise companies are all over America and are owned and operated by different sets of people in each locality. It's all about that local talent pool and good management—not the brand. Many times, a local family-owned company with a good longstanding community reputation is a better option than a franchise.

My experience revealed some common-sense clues about vetting agencies. In your exploratory conversations with the companies' marketing contacts, here are some issues to consider:

Learn the hourly rate the caregiver is actually paid, not the hourly rate you pay the agency. And exactly what are the caregiver's benefits? This will shed light on loyalty and incentive to actually show up for the job with a work ethic. It's just common sense. At any point you can always Google "pay rate for in-home care" to see the going rate in your area. Sometimes the most expensive agency could be the best if they are passing on the high hourly rate to your caregiver.

The agency turnover rate of their CNAs (certified nursing assistants). In my opinion, a high turnover rate means there is no loyalty to the agency. The agency will probably not tell you about their turnover rate. Besides, how would anyone really know? Here's a clue:

The agency contract we signed contained a clause that was downplayed. If we hired one of their CNAs privately, we had to pay the agency $10,000. That was a clue that their CNAs could easily leave for better pay and probably had no loyalty, no financial benefits to keep them interested in staying with the agency. The reason a CNA will want private work instead of agency work is that they'd like to earn a decent living with a higher hourly rate. My caregivers were paid $9 an hour, while I paid $20 an hour to the agency. They would just not show up for work in many cases, or fall asleep in a living room chair because they had just finished a night shift to make ends meet. If the agency has financial incentives, a good hourly rate, health insurance, paid vacations, training for higher levels of care or more, the caregivers have incentives to stay and do well with their agency.

What exactly does the training of the caregiver entail? Not all certified nursing assistants are the same. I found our caregivers were not CNAs. Instead, they had two hours of online video training and could not even do the basics, like scramble eggs or make a bed. Get specific about the experience and training of the agency's caregivers.

There came a time when Rick began to quickly go downhill, losing serious weight and needing to go to the ER for recurring pneumonia and eventually respiratory failure. (We didn't know it at the time, but the cancer had spread to his kidney and to his spine. Perhaps this contributed to his rapid downturn.) I needed the in-home caregivers to overlap with me, and they didn't show up, or the agency didn't have a good pool of skilled workers to draw from. Even though we had an abundance of long-term-care insurance to cover care for Rick at home, it didn't matter, because the in-home caregiver agency had such a hard time providing good workers.

In my opinion, good in-home care comes from the dedication of the "boots on the ground" like every other caregiver. The better the training and incentive for workers, the better the pool of talent from which to draw the best personality matches.

CHAPTER TEN

Hospice and the End of Life Experience

December 11, 2018, Savannah Memorial Hospital.

It was around 1 a.m. Rick was very ill, and his critical care physician at Savannah Memorial Hospital phoned me to come right away. Rick had been calling out for me, and they couldn't say how much time he had.

I got out of bed and drove the back roads from our home in Palmetto Bluff to Savannah heading south on US 17, marsh on each side of the road approaching the Talmadge Memorial Bridge. The night was so pitch black that my high beams seemed to hardly pierce the darkness.

I didn't know how long Rick could hold on. Straining to focus on the road, I remembered whispering to Rick months earlier, "Wild horses couldn't drag me away from you ... "

When I arrived, Rick's eyes were closed. But he was pulling at his hospital gown and struggling. I placed his hands on my body to comfort him as he struggled, and I quietly spoke to him. "Rick, I'm here. I'm here, my sweetheart. I'm right here with you. It's okay, I'm right here."

He was experiencing respiratory failure, the doctors told me, and we agreed that a ventilator was not only inhumane, but it was also against Rick's wishes, as expressed in his health care directives. To help him breathe, they suggested a BiPAP—which is a mask, not intubation—and I agreed so he could get some oxygen. It was too much to see him struggle.

He was moved to another room later that night.

I called Kelly and Stephen in Raleigh at 3 a.m. on December 11. It was time for everyone to come to Rick's bedside. They called the other children and Rick's lifelong friends while driving the five hours from Raleigh to Savannah Memorial Hospital.

It was late morning now. Rick was skeletal, but he was awake and eating a grape popsicle. His eyes were clear. He would fall asleep for several minutes at a time and would occasionally call out for me.

Our daughter Kelly and I were in his hospital room. It had a pleasant wall of windows and a sunny view. He was not in pain, and deep down we were in denial that Rick would die soon, nor did the physicians say that he would.

His eyes closed, and he appeared to drift off. He would raise his arms toward the ceiling and tall windows. His arms trembled, but he would straighten his back and try to reach further. His frail body and weakness did not stop him from reaching out.

We were deeply saddened to see our big, strong Rick starving and emaciated. Desperate, I asked Dr. Gard, our hospitalist, if Rick could have a feeding tube like he'd had after surgery, hoping it would give him the strength to overcome this setback. The doctors gathered to explain to me why that would not be a good idea. It would do more harm than good. Still, none of the doctors said he was dying.

Nobody mentioned having hospice come speak with our family, and I didn't know enough to ask for a hospice representative. Again, a BiPAP mask that night to keep him alive...

December 12, 2018.

The next morning, our daughter Kelly, her husband Stephen and Rick's granddaughter Sarah, all in their twenties, arrived in Rick's new room. He had a wound on the bridge of his nose from the BiPAP the night before, but he was awake and engaging. Kelly told me, "He looked and acted a hundred years old," but he spent 45 minutes chatting with his Millennials, teasing and just being himself. He'd fought his way through the night to have this time with them. It was his gift.

When I arrived with our older daughter Carolyn, Rick was losing energy and could barely be heard. He greeted me with a soft, "I love you," followed by, "Where's Carolyn?" She took his hand, and they had their private moments together. Rick had raised Carolyn, my daughter from a previous marriage, since she was five years old. He loved her as his own, and she loved him.

My moment came a few minutes later. "Hello, my knight in shining armor," I whispered. Our children were watching as a smile lit up his emaciated face.

I retrieved his wedding band from my bag. "I'd better put this on your finger to let everyone know you're taken," I told him as I slipped it onto his ring finger. It was much too big for him now. He closed his eyes, very weak, but he was still listening. "I love you," I whispered again.

Dr. Gard came into the room. We were all there—Kelly, Stephen, Sarah, Carolyn and me. Dr. Gard stood at the foot of Rick's bed and told us he felt we should now move into the hospice service.

I leaned over to Rick and asked, "Do you want any more treatment? More oxygen treatment?"

"No!" he called out as loudly as his shadow could.

I turned back to Dr. Gard. "There you have it. Rick doesn't want more treatment, and I have his health care directives. So, we all agree to go into hospice."

Dr. Gard, a gentle bear of a man, stood there looking at all of us and began to weep. We were all touched, having never seen a physician weep like this before. Later I asked Dr. Gard why he had been moved to tears. He explained that it was a combination of things, but mostly he was touched by all the young adults in the room who were there for Rick. It was unusual, he explained, for a family to lovingly move into hospice, all in agreement and supportive of the patient's best interest. He told me that too often, patients have no one at all by their bedside, or have family who put their own wishes ahead of the patient's. He was saddened that he couldn't help Rick overcome the setback and live longer.

"You were good advocates," Dr. Gard said, and then added, "I probably would have really liked Rick."

And there it was. The "white coat," the "boots on the ground," revealed as a hardworking, compassionate healer, and a wonderful human being. A hero.

A Catholic priest was called to give Last Rites. The hospice nurses advised us to go home, sleep for a few hours and come back in the morning. The process could take several days we were told.

December 13, 2018.

Carolyn, Kelly, Stephen, Sarah and I arrived as a group early the next morning. Rick's lifelong friends Tom and Joy Jackson arrived an hour or so later.

Rick had a pain medication patch and looked to be sound asleep. His breathing was very shallow: Rick was lingering for us. The doctor told us Rick could hear us. Hearing is the last sense to go, he said. A hospital chaplain guided us in our last words to Rick... "I love you... Thank you... I forgive you... Please forgive me..."

We all stood around Rick's bed touching him and even, for a moment, chatting as if we were gathered in our kitchen. The Millennials tuned in an iPhone to Rick's favorite music, the Eagles and Motown.

The usual glass half-filled with water and a small sponge were at Rick's bedside. Even though he couldn't swallow, I could still dab water on his lips. When I touched his mouth with the soaked sponge, he pursed his lips, soothed.

Tom and Joy were the first to say their private goodbyes to Rick, then left us. Thank God for them and their friendship.

Zack and Kim Taylor, our son-in-law Stephen's parents, sent a beautiful letter, which Stephen read aloud to Rick. Rick's estranged daughter, Karri—from a previous marriage —texted a message of love, which I read to him. He heard every word.

As we prepared for what was to come, each of Rick's loved ones in the room stood close to him, touching him and saying their good-byes. Love ... gratitude ... forgiveness ...

Kelly said to her father, "It's okay to go to Heaven, Dad. We're going to be okay."

Then at last came my turn. I held Rick and spoke softly.

"Love of my life, you've provided for my every desire... family, friendship, home, a wonderful life. Please forgive me if I've ever hurt you. You've done nothing to be forgiven. I love you. Now it's time for you to go to Heaven. We'll take care of one another. Your mom and dad and brother are waiting for you."

As I spoke those words, we watched Rick's spirit leave his body until the physical shell that remained didn't even resemble the man we knew.

It was just past noon. 12:26 p.m.

The room was full of supernatural love and forgiveness. It was beautiful. We were sad and happy at the same time. Rick was no longer suffering.

Much later I talked with our daughter Carolyn about how she felt during that experience, and about her lasting memories. To paraphrase Carolyn, the hardest part was the night before he died, not knowing how things would go. She felt "fortunate" and realized he had embraced us. It was "incredibly beneficial" that we were all present, having time to focus on him and say our goodbyes, comfort him and say, 'I love you.' Everything else was irrelevant."

Of the moment Rick passed, Carolyn described the feeling as bittersweet—relief that Rick was no longer burdened. The feeling was of closure. This was "exactly the way it should be. Peaceful." Seeing us all gathered around Rick strengthened her sense of family and confirmed that loved ones are of the most importance.

God's gifts of mercy, love and peace on full display.

That evening I slept in our bed at home and had a vivid dream. Rick was sitting sideways on the bed next to me, talking to me, as he often did. I recognized the line of his jaw, his shoulders, his profile. His body was no longer emaciated but healthy, his shoulders, arms and chest strong again, as I remembered him when we first met 34 years ago.

In the intimate, loving voice that he used only with me, the voice I'd heard since the day we met, he said, "Well, Kim Norris, where have you been? I've been texting and texting you." The sentiment was definitely Rick, teasing me that, as usual, he was waiting for me. The voice was Rick's. The charm of his banter was Rick. Without a doubt, he was happy and where he belonged, and he was waiting for me.

Just one little thing ... My husband had been bald the entire 34 years we were together, and it was a source of occasional good-natured teasing by his guy friends for much of his adult life. But in my "dream," he had a full head of dark hair! It still makes me smile. He must be in Heaven!

Hospice

We all did our very best as advocates for Rick. But I can't help thinking that perhaps if we had engaged hospice service sooner, we may have had more time to be together in peace—especially considering the endless ER visits, each involving six to 12 hours waiting to be seen, or ending up hospitalized for a few days but never really getting better, only to have to go back to the emergency room every week or so.

Here's what I learned in a long conversation with Sandra Bond, who was at the time the executive director of Compassus in South Carolina. With this insight, you'll be more informed than I was about how hospice service works:

Hospice is a continuation of the care service line, just like physical, occupational and speech therapy, and home health care. Hospice is about "quality of life" vs. "quantity of life." Hospice will forego all curative and heroic measures so the patient can live their life until they die a natural death from the disease process. The treatment is for symptoms, not to cure the disease.

After his battle to recover from surgery, Rick was able one afternoon to do what he loved and had longed for in those days at Duke—to take his victory walk to the dock, sit with me and just enjoy the peaceful May River off Palmetto Bluff.

But there comes a time when fighting becomes all-consuming and a cruel, losing battle. Hard as it is to admit, we can't beat death when it turns into a freight train heading straight at us. That's where hospice comes in.

According to Sandra Bond, people generally tend to wait much too long for hospice services. The reason for this is because, like myself, we don't truly understand what hospice is and the services they provide to the patient and their circle of caregivers. Hospice requires patients to meet eligibility and criteria in order to be under the hospice service line. Criteria is determined by the hospice agency. You have to ask for a referral to hospice. Like us, many people tend not to think about hospice as an alternative to care, especially while they're fighting. I didn't.

The doctors will do everything possible to keep their patients alive and heal them. They'll wait until the very last minute to mention hospice. So, like everything else, the advocate has to ask for it.

Ask for a hospice representative to come talk with you and your loved one. The conversation does not mean you're ready to give up the fight at that very moment. Nobody fought harder than we did. It just means you'll understand your options when the time comes.

It's okay to talk about hospice. I wish I'd known enough to ask. Rick was about 24 hours in hospice before he died. Maybe his suffering could have been eased had we gone into hospice service earlier. Hard to know. But it's always best to consider all the options, including hospice.

I asked Sandra Bond, "What do you want the advocate to know?" Here's her paraphrased answer:

- Learn as much as possible about the disease your loved one has. To the best of your ability, find out what to expect in terms of recovery and disease progression.

- Advocate to discharge planners. Again, this is very important from a hospice perspective. As I mentioned earlier, the discharge planner will take the path of least resistance in discharging patients. Their job is to find a place that you want to be. Hospice is an option, but it requires more time and effort for the discharge planner, due to the uncomfortable conversation at times. You'll have to ask for it. Advocate for it. Request that a hospice provider come talk with you. Advocate for the service you want. Discharge planners appreciate a plan that is thought out for a patient. The planners will respond if you don't give up.

- There are four levels of hospice care: routine home care, respite care in a certified Medicare facility, continuous home care and general in-patient care provided in a hospital setting. All levels are offered by every hospice agency, and each level of care must be determined by the medical team. Check with your hospice agency on what contractual relationship they may have with local facilities. Check your health care and long-term care insurance policies for coverage. Your insurance agent or insurance provider will help you understand specifically how hospice is covered.

CHAPTER ELEVEN

Celebration of Life and Closure

When Rick passed on December 13, 2018, his body was cremated, according to his wishes. We, the immediate family, had time to digest our profound loss, rest, think through how best to celebrate Rick's life and begin to grieve in private.

We also had time to reach out to friends and family as we planned for closure that we intended to take the form of a simple, loving, dignified memorial service on January 26, 2019, three days before his seventy-second birthday.

Not every family member was welcome to be present during Rick's final hospice experience, nor were some of them invited to attend his memorial service. It's not always easy to handle family issues at times like these.

In our family, as I'm sure it is in many others, there were some people Rick didn't want to see during his hospitalization. It's okay to honor your loved one's wishes for privacy, and that extends to the memorial service or funeral.

Advocating for Rick was a long road. It began with the diagnosis and flowed continuously in a steady stream—through treatment, surgery, hospitalization, rehabilitation, home care, escalation of his illness, end-of- life care, death and his memorial service. It doesn't end until the loved one is laid to rest with dignity and closure. I had to stay the course and advocate until the very last moment.

Upholding Rick's wishes made the final chapter of his passing dignified and respectful for all those who attended the memorial service in the spirit of love.

Rick had instructed me not to get "caught up in unnecessary funeral expenses." I realized as we planned his service that he was right. His request for cremation was best. We'd been there for Rick's final moment and watched his spirit leave his body, and the physical form that remained was nearly unrecognizable. We knew in our hearts that we wanted to return his ashes to the Earth.

We were new members of Christ Church in Savannah, thanks to our dear friends Michael Franck and Will Miller. The Reverend Michael S. White was the memorial service officiant. It was a sparkling South Carolina day in January, as sixty people from every important stage of Rick's life gathered in a small, low-country chapel, lovely in its simplicity, overlooking the May River.

Michael White guided us through a loving and dignified service. Two female Navy honor guards—perfect for a man who, with devotion, had headed a house full of women—delivered a flawless tribute, one playing "Taps" on a brass bugle. Then came the ceremonial folding of the American flag and its presentation to our family "on behalf of the President of the United States, the United States Navy and a grateful nation ... "

Kelly was the only speaker. She represented our family and delivered an amazing, loving eulogy for the man who meant so much to all of us, once again in a room full of love.

Then, following the service, a few of us went out on the May River in a small boat, a good distance from Rick's favorite neighborhood dock. There we had a ceremonial spreading of Rick's ashes.

Rick loved that river, and that dock was the symbol of his victory in his fight to come home to us.

SPEAKING OF CLOSURE

By now you know about the important role Dr. Thomas D'Amico played in our lives and the Rick's surgery at Duke University Medical Center. Rick was incredibly fortunate to have found Dr. D'Amico.

During my husband's eight weeks in the ICU, Dr. D'Amico, as busy as his schedule was, would sometimes appear silently, in the darkened ICU or early morning hours, looking in on Rick. He was someone we could trust, someone who listened and did not dismiss us as we advocated for Rick, someone who demonstrated the very best in medical care and had assembled a brilliant team to care for Rick … It's impossible to express our gratitude.

Fast-forward to January 26, 2019, the day of Rick's memorial service. Just weeks before, our friends literally took me by the hand and led me to join Christ Church in Savannah. I was now a brand-new member and barely knew Michael White, the church rector, but he graciously agreed to officiate Rick's memorial service.

As the boat headed back to the dock after the ceremonial spreading of my husband's ashes, I chatted with Michael White when someone mentioned Dr. D'Amico in conversation. Michael sat up a bit.

"Dr. Thomas D'Amico? Tommy D'Amico?"

To our collective surprise, Thomas D'Amico and Michael White knew one another quite well. Years earlier Dr. D'Amico had been instrumental in bringing Michael White in as rector of their church in Durham, North Carolina. We later learned that there was mutual admiration between the two men. We had no idea that the two were connected, nor did they know of our connection to one another. It was such a happy coincidence, although it felt like more than just that: It felt as if we were meant to know both men, who had lifted us up physically and spiritually.

That final connection helped me see that God had a plan for us all along, and He had been and continues to be with us every step of the way.

CHAPTER TWELVE

Take Good Care of Yourself

Give yourself the peace of mind of knowing that nothing is perfect,
and you have done your very best.

FINAL ACTS OF ADVOCACY ARE FOR YOURSELF

Rick's memorial service was over. All of our out-of-town friends and family who were there for the weekend returned to their lives. The silence was eerie—deafening. Even with the continuing love and support from the Palmetto Bluff community of friends and neighbors, and my children and other loved ones who were constantly in touch, there came a time to be alone with my thoughts and memories.

At any moment, the mind will replay the kindest, as well as the most horrific, details. I would often catch myself waiting for Rick to come home or expecting to see him as I rounded the corner to the kitchen, even though I was with him when he died.

I began to have symptoms of what could be described as "broken heart syndrome." Out of the blue, my heart would pound wildly, seemingly for no reason, with shortness of breath and noticeable chest pain, as if I feared for my life—in the middle of the night, in the middle of the day. Thinking I might have a heart issue, I saw my cardiologist, who put me on a heart monitor for a week and scheduled an MRA (magnetic resonance angiogram) to test for blockages. It was a precaution, the doctor explained. He'd just tested a recent widow, and although the test was fine, she had a heart attack anyway. My test results were normal, and I was fine.

I bring this up because some sort of health issue like this may happen to you. Your journey and experience may be completely different from mine. Regardless, the stress of advocating for a loved one takes a toll. Grieving takes a toll. My friends encouraged me to focus on my own health now. It's good advice.

Focusing on my own health encouraged me each day to keep a positive, grateful attitude and believe that things were going to get better. Life was going to be okay. I was motivated to take care of myself because I wanted to enjoy our children, and I especially did not want to squander the home and community Rick had provided so I would be safe and among friends.

- Take good care of yourself during and after your time as an advocate.

- You have done your very best for your loved one.

- We will each have a unique journey, a different story, but we all need to allow ourselves to focus on our own well-being.

CHAPTER THIRTEEN

The Culture of Partnerships

On January 20, 2020, Caroline DeLongchamps and I met in Charleston. She's a busy woman, manager of Patient and Family Centered Care at the Medical University of South Carolina (MUSC), but she was kind enough to spend time with a stranger and talk about patient advocacy.

Her entry into health care came as a result of a freak accident years earlier. During the momentary excitement of children getting off the school bus, her then-eleven-month-old son Sam went from playing in the yard to having his skull crushed under the wheel of a friend's SUV in her own driveway. In that one instant, an accident changed everything.

Sam, now a thriving young man, recovered well over the years as the result of world-class medical care he continues to receive at MUSC Children's Hospital. That experience led Caroline to volunteer at the hospital where Sam had his surgeries and treatment. Then came an invitation to serve as a volunteer on the Children's Health Patient and Family Advisory Council, leading her to her true calling.

Eventually Caroline sought out a paid position at the hospital and served as a guest services representative covering the pediatric intensive care units. Initially the staff saw her as a "patient advocate."

"There's Caroline. She's a patient advocate," she quoted them to me. "And I didn't like that term because it creates an 'us vs. them' mentality." She wanted to be a member of the PICU team.

When MUSC decided to create a patient-and-family-centered care department, Caroline was hired to lead the program.

> "Advocacy is great, and it's important, and there are things that I have done in the name of advocacy. But my department is *not* about patient advocacy. My department teaches the culture of partnerships. Partnerships between patients, care team members, providers and families. How do we work with each other rather than doing 'to' and 'for' our patients all the time?"

Caroline explained that she manages five Patient and Family Advisory Councils (PFAC). Patients, family members and care team members meet once a month to share with each other what is important to them and ultimately to improve the way care is delivered at MUSC. Her job is to put people in the room who can communicate their experience in a way that is teachable. She acknowledged that medical team members have a harder time hearing a message if it comes across as accusatory or threatening.

> "That's why I say we aren't about advocacy but about shifting the culture to partnerships. The core concepts of this work are: respect and dignity, participation, collaboration and information sharing. Those are our five core concepts, and everything I do is centered around those ideals."

Caroline told me during these advisory sessions that patients/ families most commonly want to find ways to better communicate with the care team.

"For example, bedside nurses giving shift report that includes the patient/family is an opportunity to educate the family about the patient's condition. Inviting a family member or caregiver to be present during shift report gives them the opportunity to hear this important exchange of information about their loved one, thus preparing them for discharge and caring for the patient at home."

Using the example of bedside shift change reports with patients and families, Caroline pointed out that this was neither revolutionary nor innovative.

"When we first rolled this out five years ago, there were barriers to doing this work, because nurses were not trained to give bedside report with patients and families. They need to complete the report in a timely way in order to let the outgoing nurse leave. Interruptions, for time and safety, were a major concern, so this report has historically been done outside the patient room on a computer in the hallway.

There are also barriers in the ICU because of the intense level of care and sensitive nature of conversations, particularly if patients are not in private rooms. So, it has taken years of culture change and discussion and training to talk about the benefits of doing shift report at the bedside for our patients, families and care teams."

Caroline's words speak directly to the opportunity to gain information that I so needed in my own experience, but I didn't know how to participate in shift reports.

This information sharing would have helped me understand my role in Rick's discharge, particularly from Duke to the inpatient rehabilitation hospital. As I was not educated beforehand by providers with the best information, Rick might have ended up in a nursing home instead of a great inpatient rehab. My self-guided decision to advocate for the right discharge and course of treatment, I'm convinced, helped Rick recover enough to enjoy at least a few months at home.

Caroline explained that caregivers do not want to increase stress for people or make things more burdensome, so a choice is given to participate in bedside report.

> "But we do want the benefits of doing so to be understood ... benefits for the family and patient, and for the medical care providers ..."

Thinking back to my outburst with Dr. D'Amico in the ICU... If I'd had that regular exchange of information, it would have helped me manage better and perhaps use that time to improve how we communicated with and understood each other, along with the realities at hand.

Rick's self-extubation was an exceptionally negative event for our family. What if, at the bedside information exchanges, the nurse had the time to mention the risk of potential self-extubation? Perhaps with a little coaching on how to find more information? Would that ugly event have ever happened? Would we have avoided that ripple of ferocious negative feelings that are still raw to this day? Would the nurses have been spared the stress of my disruption too?

How about my insistence, in the predawn hours, to summon that overworked surgery fellow about the awful calls I'd received that night from my delirious husband? Maybe I could have addressed that issue one day in a calm conversation during bedside report exchange of information. Perhaps I would have asked about his medication earlier. Perhaps Rick could have come back to us sooner and suffered less.

I heard myself expressing, more than once, that the doctor, physical therapist and nurses do *more*, until I thought it was their very best. Was I "advocating" or "adversarial"?

What if we could rewind my experience as an advocate and play it out in an imaginary hospital engaged in a pervasive culture of partnerships?

Starting at the beginning with pre-surgery clinic, what if I'd been given a 30-minute orientation on simple basics? A quick review of org charts describing roles and responsibilities of the different levels of physician, with nursing roles described and the clue that 90% of the time the bedside nurse can answer my questions or will find the right doctors ... and that nurses are patient advocates too!

Perhaps an org chart reviewing the ICU in general (including the "wound specialist") and with a few bullet points on ICU etiquette to spare the nurses some aggravation. One sheet of paper with simple coaching points, like how to be reached should the patient have a downturn. When best to check in for a status update during the night. How about including the contact info for that "pain management team"?

What if someone had spent a moment or two sharing information with me about ICU delirium? Something beyond dismissing it as not that important or "it will go away, and he won't remember a thing."

During Rick's nearly three-month hospitalization, how much of the physicians' and nurses' time would have been saved by the information shared in that 30-minute orientation, or shift change exchange of information? Would the ripples of negativity caused by my inexperience have been prevented? Would my trust in the medical care teams have been deeper, lessening time and energy drain for all concerned?

I've heard medical care professionals—brilliant, talented, driven to do their very best—talk about the complexity and constraints in hospitalization unseen by the family advocate. "You can't see the bigger picture," they'd say.

But what if we were given the option to see that bigger picture sometimes, or at least have information shared with us on a regular basis? Aren't those who are consistently informed better able to make sense of what's happening to their loved ones? Wouldn't respect, dignity, participation, collaboration and information-sharing lead to better health care, along with more time with and support for our loved ones and patients?

It's time to empower the bedside advocate to become more helpful. We need to be included in information-sharing, not just shouldering the burden to grasp at asking the right questions. With coaching, we'll have the tools to be more constructive and helpful for our loved ones and for our medical care teams.

So, good for Caroline and her mission to create a culture of partnerships anywhere medical care is delivered. I hope every single one of us will *advocate* for partnerships of this kind, whether by word of mouth, or by carefully asking our medical caregivers what kind of patient-and-family-centered care initiatives are present in their own practice or hospital.

The white coats could use our support as they try to figure out how to take control of the electronic medical records problem and find their way back to spending more time treating patients instead of "treating the computer screen."

Until that culture shift happens, I say bedside advocates have an important role to play. Maybe we can help to offset some of the burnout the white coats are experiencing as a result of being overwhelmed by the chaos, stress and time deprivation.

Why else would physicians have the highest suicide rate of any profession, and nurses have burnout rates at alarming numbers, if not that something has to give in our health care system? Sounds like patient-and-family-centered care within a culture of partnerships, less time spent on the computer and more time spent with patients could mean better health care for everyone.

As the good doctor Paul Speicher, with his kind and wide-open expression, reminds us, *"We are all in this together."*

I hope this book has shed some light and given perspective and information, and that it will be helpful to all who have taken the time to read it. Most of all, when the time has come for you to be an advocate, I hope it will reassure you when you need it most that *you're not alone.*

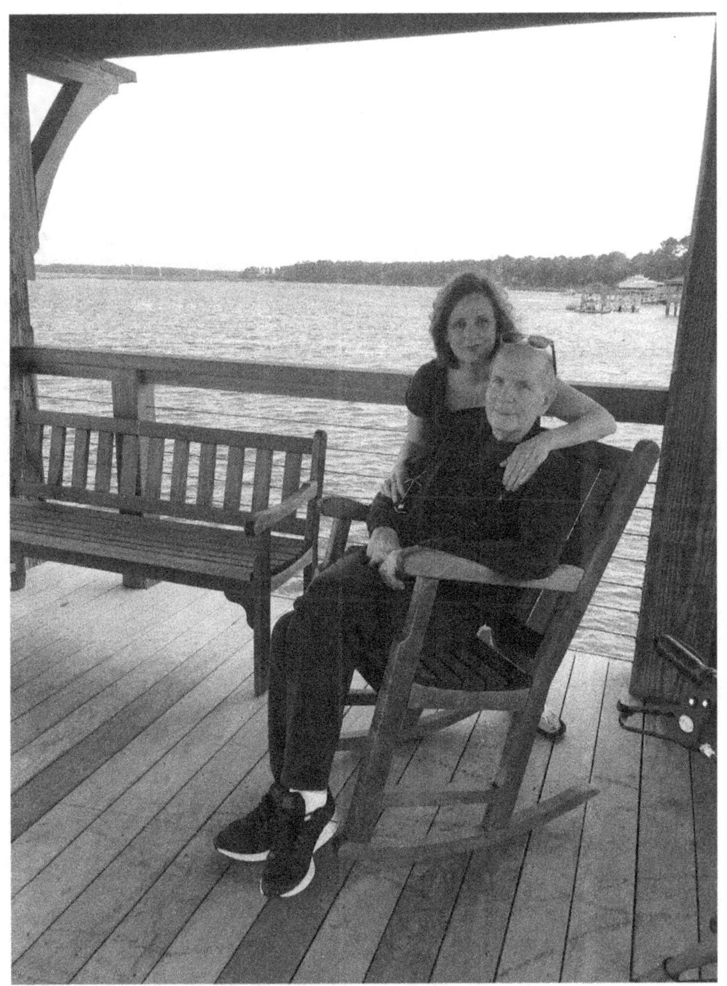

Victory, September 26, 2018

Acknowledgements

This book is truly a labor of love in honor of my husband, Rick Norris, who fought so hard to stay with us. I owe an enormous debt of gratitude to the health care professionals who generously gave of their time to share invaluable information, insight and perspective. They have my eternal gratitude for their support of this effort to help the bedside advocate.

On behalf of myself and my family, I thank them from the bottom of my heart. May God bless each and every one.

Thomas A. D'Amico MD
Gary Hock Endowed Professor of Surgery
Chief, Section of General Thoracic Surgery
Program Director, Thoracic Surgery
Duke University Medical Center
Durham, North Carolina

Paul J. Speicher, MD, MHS
Huntsville Cardiothoracic Surgeons
Huntsville, Alabama

Bethlehem Peters, RN, BSN
Cardiothoracic Intensive Care Unit
Duke University Medical Center
Durham, North Carolina
(As I write this, Bethlehem has moved on to a visiting nurse role
at Massachusetts General Hospital.)

S. Scott Balderson, PA-C
Section of General Thoracic Surgery
Duke University Medical Center
Durham, North Carolina

Dwayne Gard, MD
Chief Hospitalist - Sound Physicians
Adult Hospital Medicine - Memorial Health
Savannah, Georgia

Danielle Ofri, MD, PhD, D Litt (Hon), FACP
Bellevue Hospital
NYU School of Medicine
Editor-in-Chief, Bellevue Literary Review
New York, New York

Thomas V. Mincheff, MD, FACS
Hartsville Surgical Center
Hartsville, South Carolina

Sarah Avery
Director, Duke Health News Office
Duke University
Durham, North Carolina

Caroline DeLongchamps
Manager, Patient-and Family–Centered Care
Quality and Safety
MUSC Health, Charleston, SC

Renee Bannon, RN, BSN
Business Development Director
Encompass In-Patient Rehabilitation Hospital
Bluffton, South Carolina

Sandra Bond, RN MBA MHA
Compassus Hospice Executive Director
Savannah, Georgia/Ridgeland, South Carolina
(As I write this, Sandra is working as a private nurse)

Darlene McLeod, RNC-MNN, BSN, MPH
Much love to my friend Darlene, the accomplished nurse who coached me from afar by phone and talked me through the hospital and ICU system. I can still hear your steady voice guiding me, Darlene, making sense of the chaos, helping me advocate for Rick. God bless you.

Thank you to the business professionals in our life who lifted us up: Jeffrey Harrison, CPA, Millburn, NJ; Harriet Donnelly, e5Marketing, Basking Ridge, NJ; Robert Arundell, Esq., Hilton Head Island, SC; Robert Dempsey, Esq., Summit, NJ; Paul Pilone, LTC Global.

A huge thank-you to Justin Kovalsky, Assistant Director of Editorial Services, Johns Hopkins Medicine. The kind, patient and talented copy editor who was, in fact, my "last line of defense." I'm beyond fortunate, blessed in fact, to have had Justin on my team.

TO OUR COMMUNITY NEAR AND FAR

First and foremost, our deep love and gratitude to Tom and Joy Jackson, Rick's lifelong friends. They came multiple times throughout 2018 on a moment's notice to be at Rick's side until the end of his life. Their comforting presence lifted all of us up. They are the truest of friends.

The Raleigh millennials of Imago Dei Church... my deepest appreciation for your support, your dinners and prayers. The world is a better place because of you.

To the Rev. Michael S. White, Rector of Christ Church, Savannah, GA, thank you for your generosity and guidance.

Gratitude for our Palmetto Bluff community filled with uplifting friends and neighbors. Ann Smith Finn, for her recommendations and insight. Gratitude to Carol and Frank Riddick, Cynthia and Rick Gross, Bryan Byrne, the prayer groups and Palmetto Bluff management who were so helpful.

A special note of gratitude to my beautiful and gifted friend Gro Frivoll for her design of the book cover and the interior. Her cover design is especially dear because it captures that the call to bedside advocacy arises from love. So blessed to have Gro on my team.

Special love to the Warrior Angels of The Point, Michael Franck, William Smith III, Stan and Erin Pennington, Charlie and Dianne Russ, the late Jan Spears and husband George, Lucy and Phil Livingston, Chris and Scott Dalton, Lisa Legge and Sue Burden, all of whom sent a wave of kindness that made us feel loved.

I am especially proud of our children Kelly and Stephen Taylor, Carolyn Gamberoni and grand daughter, Sarah Sandbach. Each and every one creates a unique well of gratitude in my soul. During our 2018 ordeal, their unfailing compassion and strength was not just uplifting... it was the definition of love. Every parent dreams of such children. Rick and I were extraordinarily blessed to have their wings around us when we needed them. Rick lived to see what wonderful adults they've all become, and for that I am truly grateful.

A special thanks to Hillary B. Smith, my incredible friend who showed up to give support, hope and love throughout the worst of times.

And to Lindsay Harrison, talented author, professional advisor, and my writing coach whose encouragement gave me the confidence to keep writing through my grief, and made this labor of love possible.

REFERENCES

Definition of "Advocate": *Easton's Bible Dictionary*

Definition of "Advocatus": *WordSense Dictionary*

Chapter One:

Source: Census Bureau's Vintage Population Estimates.

Source: *US population with a hospitalization 2000-2018 by age.* Published by Statista Research Department, May 27, 2021

Source: *Total hospitals number U.S. 1975-2019* www.statista.com

Chapter Four:

Definition of nocebo effect: Merriam-Webster Dictionary. "Doctors, Nurses and the Paperwork Crisis That Could Unite Them": *New York Times*, article by Theresa Brown and Stephen Berman, published December 31, 2019.

Medscape National Physician Burnout, Depression & Suicide Report, 2019, www.medscape.com/slideshow/2019-lifestyle-burnout-depression-6011056.

"Physicians Experience Highest Suicide Rate of Any Profession," Pauline Anderson, May 7, 2018, www.medscape.com/viewarticle/896257.

"The Business of Health Care Depends on Exploiting Doctors and Nurses. One Resource Seems Infinite and Free: The Professionalism of Caregivers": *New York Times*, article by Dr. Danielle Ofri, June 8, 2018.

"The Medical Hierarchy - Defining Medical Terms" chart, and "The Nursing Hierarchy – Defining Nursing Team Members" chart courtesy of: The Empowered Patient®, Guide to Hospital Care for Patients and Families, ©2009 Dr. Julia A. Hallisy and Helen W. Haskell, Updated 2012 Dr. Julia A. Hallisy, An Empowered Patient® Publication.

Chapter Five:

Definition of tracheostomy: Merriam-Webster Dictionary.

"Self-Extubation in ICU Patients," by Davitha Selvan BS, Hawa Edriss MD, Mark Sigler MD, Jim Tseng BS. The Southwest Respiratory and Critical Care Chronicles, published electronically, 10/15/2014. SWRCCC 2014; 2(8): 31-34, doi: 10.12746/swrccc2014.0208.100.

REFERENCES

Chapter Six:

Definition of "step-down unit": *Farlex Partner Medical Dictionary*, Farlex 2012.

"Delirium in the Intensive Care Unit," www.ncbi.nlm.nih.gov/pmc/articles/PMC2391269, by Timothy D. Girard, Patrik P. Pandharipande, and E. Wesley Ely; Crit Care 2008; 12(Suppl 3): S3. Published online May 14, 2008. doi: 10.1186/cc6149. This article is part of *Critical Care* Volume 12 Supplement 3: Analgesia and sedation in the ICU. Full contents of the supplement are available online at http://ccforum.com/supplements/12/S3.

"New center formed to treat, study ICU delirium, dementia," by Nancy Humphrey, VUMC Reporter, October 4, 2018. https://news.vumc.org/2018/10/04/new-center-formed-to-treat-study-icu-delirium-dementia.

"Hospitals struggle to address terrifying and long-lasting 'ICU delirium'," by Usha Lee McFarling, October 14, 2016. www.statnewscom/2016/10/14/icu-delirium-hospitals/.

Chapter Seven:

The Four Seasons Poems, a Borzoi Book published by Alfred A. Knopf. This selection by J.D. McLatchy first published in Everyman's Library, 2008.

"Desperado" written by Donald Hugh Henley, Glenn Lewis Frey.

Chapter Eight:

"Value of Inpatient Rehabilitation Hospital Care Reaffirmed," Center for Medicare Advocacy, May 17, 2016, T. Edelman, Center for Medicare Advocacy
www.medicareadvocacy.org/
value-of-inpatient-rehabilitation-hospital-care-reaffirmed/.

Chapter Thirteen:

Patient- and Family-Centered Care, Medical University of South Carolina, muschealth.org/patients-visitors/about-us/ quality-and-safety/pfcc.

Institute for Patient- and Family-Centered Care, 6917 Arlington Road, Suite 309, Bethesda, MD 20814, https://www.ipfcc.org/ about/pfcc.html.

APPENDIX

Figure 1

The Medical Hierarchy - Defining Medical Teams

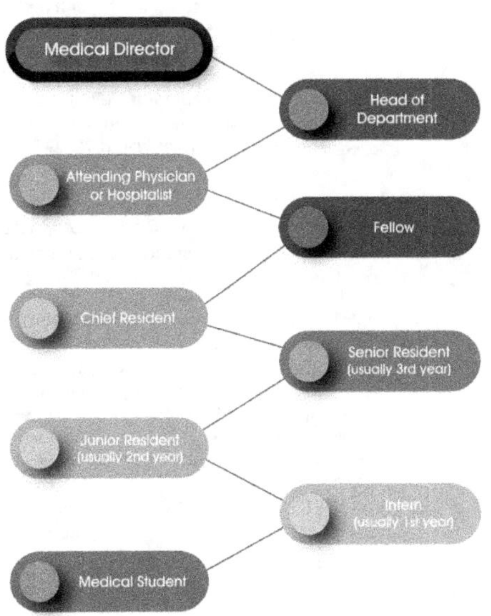

MEDICAL DIRECTORS are physician leaders who oversee all the staff physicians on staff. Medical directors coordinate all aspects of both inpatient and outpatient care in hospitals and work to establish institutional policies and practices that will ensure high quality care to patients. All of your physicians ultimately answer to the medical director.

Your attending is the doctor ultimately responsible for your treatment plan. If you cannot get the help you need from the attending you can ask to speak to the **HEAD OF THE DEPARTMENT** he is associated with, such as orthopedics, cardiology, etc.

ATTENDING PHYSICIANS are the most senior doctors directly responsible for your medical decision-making and treatment while you are in the hospital. Attending physicians are fully trained doctors who have completed a minimum of three years of residency training and who may have passed a board examination in a specialty. Collectively, the attending physicians treating patients at a hospital are called the **Medical Staff.**

HOSPITALISTS are physicians who focus solely on the care of hospitalized patients. They are usually employed either by the hospital or by a medical group that contracts with the hospital. In some hospitals, hospitalists take over responsibility from your regular doctor when you enter the hospital and function as your attending physician. In others, they serve as a backup to your attending physician. You should inquire if your hospital employs hospitalists so you will know what to expect if you are admitted. Call the patient relations department or the admitting office to obtain this information.

House Staff is a generalized term used by hospitals to cover doctors- in-training, or residents, who may range from interns just out of medical school to fellows with years of experience. In teaching hospitals, house staff will direct a great deal of your medical treatments. Find out if your local hospital is a teaching hospital so you will be prepared to interact with residents. The following are different levels of house staff you may encounter.

FELLOWS operate at a level of responsibility just below attending physicians. They are physicians who have completed their primary residency and have chosen to pursue advanced training (a fellowship) in a particular specialty. Fellows may have little direct patient contact and it may not be obvious that a fellow is participating in your treatment. Be sure to ask, since fellows, like other residents, can write orders in your chart and make decisions about your treatment plan.

RESIDENTS have graduated from medical or osteopathic school and passed a national licensing exam. A resident is a licensed "MD" (osteopaths are called "DO") but he cannot work without supervision until he has completed a minimum of three years of hands-on training (the primary residency). The **CHIEF RESIDENT** is a senior resident who directs the activities of other residents and functions as their immediate "boss." Just below the Chief Resident is the **SENIOR RESIDENT** (usually a third year resident) and below them are **JUNIOR RESIDENTS** (usually in their second year). These are the basic categories - some residency programs in specialty fields can be as long as eight years.

INTERNS are doctors who have completed medical school and are in their first year of residency training. Some hospitals do not use the term "intern" and instead refer to interns as first year residents, R-1 's or PGY-1 's (for Postgraduate year 1). Regardless of the name used, interns have a medical degree but are not yet licensed to practice medicine on their own, which requires them to be supervised by senior MDs or DOs.

The Nursing Hierarchy - Defining Nursing Team Members

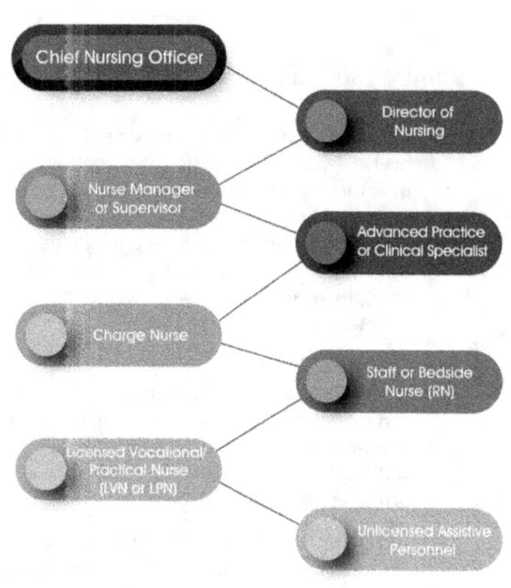

REGISTERED NURSES (RNs) comprise the largest segment of healthcare workers. Because they are the most hands-on of all hospital caregivers, the bedside nurse may be an important advocate for you. Registered nurses have a bachelor's degree (BSN), an associate degree (ADN), or a diploma from an approved nursing program.

Nurses spend a great deal of their time providing direct patient care. Your bedside nurse is continuously observing, monitoring, and assessing your progress and may detect the first signs of a complication. If and when a nurse notes a sudden or subtle change in your condition, he or she initiates an appropriate response such as providing nausea medication or calling the doctor to come to the bedside.

NURSING SUPERVISORS and **NURSE MANAGERS** are part of the leadership team and are considered "nursing executives." There is a nurse manager or nurse supervisor available 24 hours a day who is the direct supervisor of the charge nurses. A nurse manager or supervisor should be available to patients, either in person or via consultation in an on-call capacity. Nursing supervisors are overseen by a **DIRECTOR OF NURSING** or a **CHIEF NURSING OFFICER (CNO)**.

ADVANCED PRACTICE NURSES are registered nurses who have completed advanced training beyond the basic criteria that all RNs must fulfill. They meet higher educational and clinical requirements than other nursing groups. Within this category, there are two groups:

- **NURSE PRACTITIONERS** work closely with physicians and are qualified to diagnose and treat common illnesses and injuries. An NP can actually function as a patient's main healthcare provider.
- A **CLINICAL NURSE SPECIALIST** functions as an expert whose focus is on a specific area of nursing practice. For example, a CNS may specialize in treating surgical, diabetic, geriatric, cardiovascular, psychiatric or pediatric patients.

CHARGE NURSES are responsible for scheduling and directing the nursing care in a specific ward or unit during each assigned shift. The charge nurse is the first person to contact if there is a problem with your bedside nurse. If you are not satisfied with her response, ask to speak to the nurse manager.

STAFF NURSES are registered nurses who provide direct patient care at the bedside. Your staff nurse will be up-to-date on your vital signs, medications, and overall treatment plan. Your bedside nurse is the first nurse to consult if you have a question or concern. Not all members of the nursing staff have RN degrees. Patients are often cared for by licensed vocational nurses (LVNs or LPNs) and by assistive personnel such as nurses' aides (NAs) and patient care assistants (PCAs).

A **LICENSED VOCATIONAL NURSE OR LICENSED PRACTICAL NURSE (LVN or LPN)** completes 1500 hours or approximately one year of training and is licensed by the state in which he or she works. In general, LVNs perform basic patient duties such as taking vital signs, monitoring IV's and other catheters, administering oral medications and writing notes in the patient's chart. LVNs collect patient information but they do not make treatment decisions based on these facts, since this requires the training and skill of a registered nurse.

ASSISTIVE PERSONNEL are individuals who work in a supportive role under a licensed nurse. Assistants have duties such as helping patients with their basic needs, answering call lights and taking vital signs. Some assistive personnel, including nurses' aides (NAs) and nursing assistants may be licensed by their states but other types of workers such as patient care assistants (PCAs) may have brief training courses that do not require passing a state licensing exam.